Radiology of the Spine

Editor
A. Wackenheim, Strasbourg

Jean-Claude Dosch

Trauma

Conventional Radiological Study
in Spine Injury

With 154 Figures

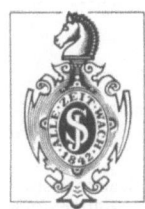

Springer-Verlag
Berlin Heidelberg New York Tokyo 1985

Dr. Jean-Claude Dosch

Service de Radiologie
Centre de Traumatologie et d'Orthopédie
de Strasbourg
10, Avenue A. Baumann
F-67400 Illkirch-Graffenstaden

ISBN-13: 978-3-642-45582-7   e-ISBN-13: 978-3-642-45580-3
DOI: 10.1007/978-3-642-45580-3

Library of Congress Cataloging in Publication Data. Dosch, J.-C. (Jean-Claude), 1946-. Trauma. (Radiology of the spine ; v. 1) Bibliography: p. Includes index. 1. Spine–Wounds and injuries–Diagnosis. 2. Spine–Radiography. 3. Diagnosis, Radioscopic. I. Title. II. Series.   RD533.D67   1984   617'.375   84-20315
ISBN-13: 978-3-642-45582-7

© by Springer-Verlag Berlin Heidelberg 1985
Softcover reprint of the hardcover 1st edition 1985

Reproduction of the figures: Gustav Dreher GmbH, Stuttgart

2127/3130-543210

*„L'image est souveraine
le langage est servile”*

Foreword

Progress in traumatology of the vertebral spine has been restrained for a long time by two hindering factors. The first obstacle is presented by the differences in approach and a conflict of competences. The neurosurgeons, considering only the spinal chord, have confined themselves to indications for laminectomy, an insufficient and usually ineffective intervention. The orthopedic surgeons, on the other hand, obsessed by the fear of medullary lesions, have long hesitated to apply the fundamental rules for the treatment of fractures, namely precise reduction followed by strict immobilization, thus depriving themselves of the efficacy of radiculomedullar decompression and of the protection this procedure affords to these structures when they are themselves involved in the trauma.

Taking these facts into account, together with the rather poor results of laminectomy, the specialists have wisely and successfully recommended that one should abstain from treating the initial lesion, but rather attenuate the damage by appropiate nursing care and adequate reeducation.

The second hindering factor was the insufficient knowledge of the extreme complexity of the anatomic lesions. This explains the orthopedists' relative caution; one only treats well what one knows well.

More precise analysis of the lesions, not only of the bones but also of the joints, i.e., the osteofibrous involvement, is mainly based on strict radiologic semiology, which is rendered difficult because these structures are simultaneously affected.

We are greatly indebted to Dr. DOSCH, radiologist at our Center, for having undertaken this difficult task, using all available conventional radiologic techniques.

The results of his efforts are presented here. The reader will appreciate his careful analysis and precise deductions as well as the excellent quality of the illustrations.

The value of this book is enhanced by the taking into account of the recent major contribution made by CT investigations of the vertebral column, permitting the realization of an old dream, the visualization of the vertebra and its lesions in transverse section. This in no way lessens the value of the two standard projections, but supplements them. Contemporary traumatologists are grateful to have at their disposal, thanks to the efforts of their radiologist colleagues, imaging of a precision never realized before, allowing them to base their diagnosis and therapeutic procedures on anatomical data of indisputable validity. Dr. DOSCH is to be congratulated on his work.

Professor IVAN KEMPF
Chairman and Medical Director

Dr. ARSENE GROSSE
Chief of Department of Emergency
and Neurotraumatologic Surgery

Center for Traumatology and Orthopedics Strasbourg

Prefaces

My student and friend, Dr. J. C. Dosch, who is now chief of a Department of Radiotraumatology in Strasbourg, has had the great privilege of authoring the first of a series of books devoted to radiology of the spine. I have no hesitation in saying that spinal radiodiagnosis is a speciality of Strasbourg: the books and works of Drs. Elisabeth Babin and Pierre Capesius have set the scene for J. C. Dosch's contribution in this field. After several years' collaboration with Prof. Y. Kempf, Dr. R. Raber and Dr. M. Dupuis, J. C. Dosch has achieved a very high level of competence in the imaging of the vertebral spine. This competence has given him the courage and the right to question what was regarded as established, to criticize what was generally accepted, and to demonstrate that certain beliefs must be abandoned.

In this first work J. C. Dosch teaches us how to review the whole roentgenographic semantics in spinal traumatology. The radiologic images of injured vertebrate, their structural integration in their originating segment, and the extraction of therapeutic indications are presented, often from a completely fresh point of view.

J. C. Dosch's analysis is made with a precision that may, at first sight, seem excessive to a reader who is not a specialist in radiotraumatology. The author proceeds to the analysis in two very distinct steps, as befits one who has studied in Strasbourg. Indeed, he knows perfectly how to differentiate between commentary, i.e., translation of the image into words, and interpretation. The latter means interpretation of the comment, and may vary with the circumstances (patient's age, family commitments, professional demands, associated diseases, therapeutic possibilities, etc.). In contrast, the commentary is immutable: it is the verbal image, whatever the context may be.

Last but not least, I would like to mention J. C. Dosch's sensitivity and warmth, which have also done much to make him one of my favorite students.

Auguste Wackenheim
Professor and Chairman of Radiology
University of Strasbourg, France

Participating in the presentation of Dr. J. C. DOSCH's remarkable work on the traumatic spine is a pleasant task, if only to underline the advances in radio-traumatology over the last 10 years. This progress is certainly due in part to the significant technological evolution that has taken place, but is also the result of constant collaboration between radiologists and surgeons which has already long been the policy at this Center for Traumatology and Orthopedics.

For a very long time radiotraumatology was the preserve of surgeons, since radiologists were not much interested in "broken bones."

It was only with the creation of centers for orthopedics and traumatology such as the one in Strasbourg that this speciality became recognized.

This remarkable and original work by Dr. DOSCH was made possible by the infrastructure of our Center, which permits real teamwork, inlcuding in particular, collaboration with the neurotraumatologist.

This work gives the basics of interpretation, which is indispensable not only to the radiologist but equally to the surgeon concerned with traumatology.

Dr. J. C. DOSCH's experience in this field is confirmed by this book, which is also remarkable in the precision of the descriptions and analysis and the richness of the illustrations, and which constitutes a true reference book and does honor to the Department of Radiology of the Center of Traumatology of Strasbourg.

> Docteur R. RABER
> Chief, Department of Radiology,
> Center for Traumatology and Orthopedics
> Strasbourg, France

I do not like to speak of my friends; even less so when they are my best friends. The author of this work is one of these, in addition to being the faithful colleague I work with every day. The task of presenting him weighs heavy, as his modesty is such that he will perhaps resent my speaking too well of him. However, it is only true say that he is an indefatigable worker; that his pursuit of knowledge is insatiable; and that he is generous in sharing this knowledge. It is true that the smallest detail excites his curiosity and ignites fresh passion.

He knows how to master each radiologic problem with a calm approach and without going to extremes, so as to give it the proper perspective in radiologic semiology.

This work is the fruit of his labor, but it also illustrates a large mass of data from our department.

He knows how to make the radiologic image speak to explain movements, mechanisms, and finally traumatism itself.

It is a pleasure to speak thus of this friend.

> Docteur MICHEL DUPUIS
> Chief, Department of Radiology,
> Center for Traumatology and Orthopedics
> Strasbourg, France

Contents

Chapter 3 Traumas of the Thoracic and Lumbar Spine

Chapter 4 Comprehensive Study

Chapter 5 Classification

Introduction

Presented for a long time as being harmful, radiologic investigation in traumatic lesions of the spine formerks consisted mostly in a very brief and thus incomplete and inadequate examination.

This was attributable in part to the surgeons' impatience, occasioned by the patients' clinical status, but also by the radiologists' misunderstanding of the mechanisms of such lesions. And these radiologic data were used to decide on the treatment!

With this book the author intend to rationalize the investigation and the interpretation of the radiologic data. As a matter of fact, we do not think that a patient with a trauma to the spine can undergo a so-called standard examination. Therefore one should always proceed to first-step radiographs, preferably taken with the patient on the transportation stretcher in the same position as on admission. These pictures are carefully examined before other radiographs. These are dependent on the possibility of active or passive mobilization of the patient.

The interpretation of the first-step radiographs is thus fundamental. It is very difficult and is based on a new form of radiosemiology depending on the variability of the image with regard to the incidence of the beam. Under these conditions the projection of the various anatomical structures, whether they are damaged or undamaged, is dictated by the incidences and projections, and the problem is similar to one of descriptive geometry.

Second-step radiologic investigation, comprising tomograms, positive contrast radiographs, and CT, is still indispensable, and we shall see later in what circumstances it is indicated.

The radiologist does not only aim at establishing a precise description of the bony, ligamentous, and/or medullar lesions however; after this analytic phase all the data should be integrated in a comprehensive study. Thus, it is for the radiologist to indicate the functional and prognostic value of each type of lesion, whether this is due to distraction, to compression, or to a transverse or rotatory shearing movement. The radiosemiological analysis must be directed at a definition of these different parameters and a decision, for each type of lesion, as to whether this is stable or unstable.

Our intention ist not to give therapeutic, orthopedic, or surgical indications, but rather to povide surgeons with the indispensable data with a view to the most suitable noninvasive means of reduction, leaving them to select the method of stabilizing the lesions.

The radiologist has, and will keep, a special place in the management of injuries to the spine. The patients' chances of recovery depend to a great extent on the quality of the radiologic investigations.

Chapter 1 Descriptive and Functional Anatomy

The vertebral column has three roles: a static and a dynamic role, and that of providing protection for the radiculomedullary axis. Three structures combine to ensure these functions, i.e., bones, disks and ligaments, and muscles. As soon as one of these structures becomes incompetent the entire set is destabilized. Therefore surgeons and radio-traumatologists should always keep this in mind and their reasoning should be a synthesis of that attributable to the anatomist, the physiologist, and the neurologist.

A. Descriptive Anatomy

I. Vertebral Body

The vertebral body has the structure of a short bone. From the embryologic point of view, the posterior arch is independent. A first ossification centers, already visible at birth, appears in the prebony cartilage of the vertebral body. A second ossification center appears around the age of 14 or 15 as an epiphyseal nucleus, which gives rise to the annular epiphyseal disk. Thus the vertebral body has a shell-like structure with dense cortical bone surrounding spongy bone. The superior and inferior aspects are referred to as the plates, the anterior aspect as the anterior wall, and the posterior aspect as the posterior wall. In its compact envelope, the spongy bone is distributed in trabeculations according to the force lines: the trabeculae are vertical, extending from the superior to the inferior plate, or horizontal, linear or circular, joining the lateral aspects, or oblique, extending between plates and walls.

A characteristic type of oblique trabeculation is constituted by fan-like fibers, demonstrating the existence of force lines between the vertebral body and the posterior arch. The trabeculations arise from the vertebral plates and head through the pedicle towards the spinous and articular processes.

The distribution of the force lines creates a weaker area in the anterior third of the vertebral body and an area of high resistance, mainly to compression forces, in the posterior third of the body including the pedicles and the posterior wall. Thus the anterior part is crushed by an axial compression of 600 kg/cm^2, whereas the posterior wall resists up to 800 kg/cm^2.

The layer of compact bone limiting the vertebral plates is perforated by numerous orifices, allowing hydrostatic pressure exchanges between the vertebral interstitial tissue and the disk. The arterial vascular foramina are located mainly on the lateral and the anterior aspects. The posterior aspect has an orifice for the exit of the veins.

The vertebral bodies vary widely in size, shape, and proportions in the different regions of the column.

1. Cervical Segment
a) First Cervical Vertebra (C1)

The first cervical vertebra differs from all other vertebrae in lacking a body; its centrum fuses with that of the axis to form the odontoid process. Disk C1–C2, which is visible up to the age of 3–4 years, constitutes the base of the odontoid process.

In some circumstances there is an absence of ossification at this level, which is seen on film as a homogeneous, harmonious, clear area, with well defined parallel margins, called a "vestigial disk": this must not be mistaken for a fracture of the odontoid process base.

The first cervical vertebra is thus somewhat ringlike. Laterally it is formed by two oval bony masses whose long axes run forward and medially, each bearing a superior articular facet facing upward and medially, and an inferior articular facet that also runs forward and medially but has an anteroposterior convexity and faces downwards and medially, which articulate with the lateral masses of the axis. The lateral masses are connected in front by a short anterior arch and at the back by a longer curved posterior arch.

b) Second Cervical Vertebra (C2)

The vertebral body of C2 has assimilated the body of C1 in its centrum. It is distinguished by a strong toothlike process, the odontoid process or dens, which juts vertically upward from the body: it articulates with the anterior arch of the atlas and serves as a pivot on which the atlas rotates.

The upper surface is flanked by a pair of large oval facets, which extend laterally from the body on the adjoining parts of the pedicles. They face upward and outward, and they are convex from front to back and plane from side to side.

The inferior aspect of the C2 body is similar to that of the other cervical vertebrae.

c) Lower Cervical Segment (C3–C7)

The bodies are smaller and roughly cubical. The posterior part of the body bears the uncinate processes, which constitute a guide or a rail for the flexion, extension, or lateroflexion movements. The superior aspect is raised laterally by two high sagittal and vertical bony lips called the uncinate processes, which face upward and medially. The inferior aspect bears two notches or facets, facing downward and laterally. These articular facets are roughened by cartilage; they constitute an articulation which is contained in a capsule limited medially by the vertebral disk. The inferior aspect of the seventh cervical vertebra does not bear uncinate facets, but has the characteristics of a thoracic vertebra.

2. Dorsal Segment

In the thoracic segment the bodies are roughly cylindrical, except that their posterior surface is concave.

The thoracic vertebrae show a gradual increase in size downward from T1 to T12. All are distinguished by costal facets on the sides of their bodies, and all but the last two by facets on their transverse processes. These articulate respectively with the heads and tubercles of the ribs.

3. Lumbar Segment

The five lumbar vertebrae differ in that they are larger. The vertebral bodies are wider from side to side, a little deeper in front, and plane behind. The fifth lumbar vertebra is markedly deeper in front than behind so that on a lateral view it has a cuneiform appearance with a wide anterior base.

II. Articular Pillars

The articular (or posterior) pillars constitute the major structure of the posterior arch. They are located between the pedicle and the lamina and comprise three distinct elements: the superior articular processes, the inferior articular processes and, between them, a bony bridge called the pars interarticularis. The site and orientation of the articular processes vary at the different vertebral levels; they adapt to the functional mobility of each segment. Together with the articular facets of the over- and underlying vertebrae they form articulations, which have a poor segmental mobility. But the overall amplitude of the movements obtained by the cumulated movements of all the posterior articular pillars is very wide and flexible.

The mobility of the posterior articular pillars works like a spring for which the energy is provided progressively at each level.

The posterior pillars have a dynamic role, in contrast to the anterior somatic pillar, which has a static role.

1. Cervical Segment

In the cervical segment the articular processes are situated posteriorly and laterally to the vertebral body, which they largely overlap. This is perfectly visible on a frontal projection, and more particularly on a DORLAND's incidence on which the vertebral body is free of any superimposition other than the laminae and spinous processes.

The articular surfaces are orientated in a plane at about 45° to the vertical plane. We thought it would be interesting to measure the orientation of the superior and inferior articular processes with reference to the homologous vertebral plates. These measurements showed that the orientation of the inferior articular facets with regard to the lower vertebral plate is relatively constant at about 47–50°. In contrast, the orientation of the superior articular facets is much more variable and can even reach 60°. There is thus an elementary angular divergence for each vertebra between the superior and inferior articular process.

These difference in the orientation of the articular gliding plane produces a lordosis of the cervical segment, which is of bony and architectural origin.

If the posterior articular interspaces of each intervertebral level are parallel, the lordosis of bony origin is equal to the sum of the elementary angular variations, i.e., theoretically equal to the angle formed by the lower vertebral plate of C2 and the upper vertebral plate of C7.

The interapophyseal articulations permit kinds of movements, i.e., flexion–extension, lateroflexion, and rotation.

During flexion movements the inferior facet of the vertebra above glides upward and forward relative to the superior facet of the underlying vertebra. Consequently there is a partial uncovering of the articular space, a superior anteroposterior interarticular space loss, and a posteroinferior gap of the same size. The gliding and angulation motion is also transmitted to the vertebral body. Thus the edge of the inferior plate of the underlying vertebra winds around the blunt edge of the upper plate of the subjacent vertebra. During extension the movements take place in the opposite direction, but are checked by the existence of a bony abutment, which is not the case for flexion movement.

The segmental amplitude of these movements is limited: we shall see the limit values allowed during the study of severe sprains.

The global amplitude of flexion is limited anatomically by the contact of the lower jaw with the sternum. The mean values are 40° for flexion and 60° for extension.

Nevertheless, and in spite of the bony abutment, purely posterior interapophyseal luxations without bone lesions are far from rare.

Three major reasons should be considered:

1) The flexion movement is accompanied by lateroflexion and rotation: in such conditions the luxation is inevitably unilateral and located on the opposite side to the lateroflexion. This mechanism occurs frequently in road accidents with lateral shock or with anteroposterior shock, the spine being in a lateroflexed rotated position in the latter case.

2) The movement is a pure flexion movement, and its entire amplitude occurs between two vertebrae. This condition is realized when a part of the lower cervical spine has become stiff, either because of a pre-existing functional block or because of contracture.

3) A very forceful shock is sustained, e.g., frontal percussion at high speed against a fixed obstacle, the entire resistance to the kinetic force being transmitted to the articulations and posterior uniting structures. This causes posterior interarticular extraction (distraction) force, which is proportional to the weight of the skull.

This is commonly seen in motorcyclists wearing crash helmets. In fact the combined weights of the skull and the helmet mean that the kinetic energy is about twice as high as at the same speed without a helmet.

Lateroflexion and rotation movements never occur in isolation, since the articular facets are not plane but convex and concave respectively. On the side of the lateroflexion the articular facet is lowered, while on the opposite side it is raised.

The mean amplitude of these movements is 20° for lateroflexion and 40–45° for rotation.

Trauma caused to the cervical spine by lateral shock have two quite distinct components:

1. A compression force acting on the side to which the head is lateroflexed or rotated, which is mainly responsible for fractures of the articular processes or of the pars interarticularis
2. A distraction force located on the opposite side, which is responsible for luxation.

2. Dorsal Segment

The posterior articular pillars are constituted mainly by the laminae, which at this level are higher than they are wide. The posterior articular facets are thin and located on the continuations of the pedicles. On its posterior aspect the superior articular process has a facet roughened with cartilage, plane or very slightly transversely convex, facing backward, upward, and slightly laterally.

The lower articular process is located on the continuation of its superior homolog on the anterior aspect of the laminae. Its articular facet has the opposite orientation, forward and medial, while transversely it is slightly concave. Moreover, it is located further back than its superior homolog. As a consequence, the cumulative effect is a physiological lordosis of bony origin.

In this segment, too, the orientation of the articular facets permits three types of movement with different degrees of freedom: flexion and extension, lateroflexion, and axial rotation.

While the total amplitude of flexion has a mean value of 35–40°, that of the extension movement is limited to 25° by two bony abutments, i.e., the accumulation of the laminae and the exaggerated obliquity of the spinous processes, between which there is a large contact area and a very restricted interspinous space.

In contrast to the lumbar segment, in the thoracic segment a relatively significant degree of rotation (35°) is possible. This is because the concave orientation of the articular interline has a large radius of curvature, the rotation center projecting forward on the vertebral body. In view of the slenderness of the superior articular processes, the architectural lordosis, and the anterior location of the center of rotation, the thoracic spine is very much exposed to constraints during the flexion and rotation movements. In traumas caused by a direct posterior shock the lesions are not due to hyperextension or hyperflexion but rather to a shearing mechanism.

3. Lumbar Segment

The lumbar posterior articular pillars are the most massive in the spine. In contrast to those of the cervical segment, they project, on a frontal view, within the limits of the vertebral body, while remaining on the same vertical line as those of the cervical vertebrae. The superior articular process is situated in the continuation of the pedicle following a plane slanting backward and to the side. Its articular facet faces backward and to the side. The inferior articular process is clearly more medial. It arises from the inferior margin of the posterior arch near the junction of the lamina with the spinous process, following a plane slanting downward and laterally. Its articular facet faces laterally and forward. The pars interarticularis is situated between the superior and inferior articular process. The

posterior articular interspace, formed by the embedding of the inferior articular process of the overlying vertebra in the superior articular process of the underlying vertebra, is backwardly concave. In contrast to that of the thoracic vertebrae, its rotation center is thus posterior, on the side of the spinous processes, and also has a small radius of curvature. The center of rotation is located progressively further back as lower vertebrae are considered. Because of its posterior situation, the lumbar intervertebral disk is subjected, to shearing forces during rotation, which restricts the amplitude of the rotation movements even further. We should like to recall that during rotation, the thoracic intervertebral disk works in axial torsion, due to the anterior location of its rotation center. This anatomical predisposition accounts for the small amplitude of the left and right rotation of the lumbar spine, which reaches hardly 10° overall.

Extension accompanied by hyperlordosis has a mean amplitude of 30°. Flexion, with its delordosing effect, has an amplitude of 40°. Different studies have shown that the widest segmental amplitude occurs between L4 and L5, that is to say at the union between a semimobile vertebra, L5, and the first mobile vertebra, i.e., L4. The left and right lateral flexion is about 25°. All these values depend of course on the age and the individual morphology of the particular patient.

III. Bony Bridges: Pedicles and Laminae

The anterior pillars are linked to the posterior pillars by bony bridges. The functional junction between the anterior and posterior pillars is made by the pedicles. The biomechanical function of the pedicles is that of a lever transmitting the forces from the vertebral body to the articular pillars and vice versa. The pedicles increase in thickness from the top downward. Thus the two last lumbar vertebrae have the most solid pedicles. Between two adjacent vertebrae the pedicles are involved in the formation of the intervertebral foramen, for which they constitute the superior and inferior limit, whereas the pillars delimit its anterior and posterior borders.

The posterior pillars are also linked to each other by the laminae, which join at the midline to provide insertion points for the spinous processes.

IV. Accessory Processes

On each vertebra there are three nonarticular processes: two lateral, paired and symmetrical, called the transverse processes, and a single median one, the spinous process.

1. Transverse

In the cervical segment the transverse processes are situated to the front, in the transverse continuation of the vertebral body. They are formed by two roots delimiting an orifice, i.e., the transverse foramen for the vertebral artery and vein.

In the thoracic segment the transverse processes are located to the outside of the articular pillars and obliquely behind; on their anterior aspect they have an articular facet that receives the costal tubercle to form the costo-transverse joint.

In the lumbar segment they are located opposite the articular pillars in a frontal plane. The morphological variations of the transverse processes are explained by the ontogenic development of the ribs.

2. Spinous

Each cervical vertebra has a short, wide, and almost horizontal spinous process with a bifid extremity. In the thoracic segment the spinous processes are markedly oblique and long, whereas in the lumbar segment they are horizontal and wide.

The biomechanical role of the accessory transverse and spinous processes is to act as insertion bases for the ligaments and muscles, which can than function like shrouds. The spinous processes also act as bony abutments to limit the extension movements and the transverse processes, to limit the lateral flexion.

V. Intervertebral Means of Union

1. Vertebral Bodies

The articulation between two vertebral bodies is provided by the adjacent vertebral plates linked by the intervertebral disk. This disk is made up of two parts: a central part, the nucleus pulposus, which is located on the midline at the junction of the median and posterior third of the vertebral body, and a peripheral part or fibrous ring around the nucleus, consisting of concentric fibrous layers. The intervertebral disk permit three basic types of movement: flexion, lateral flexion, rotation (left or right), and gliding or shearing. Resistance of the intervertebral disk to axial compression forces is good but it is less resistant to shearing forces. Vascularization of the disk allowing correct functioning of this articulation comes mainly from the vertebral body through the vertebral plates. Any traumatic lesion interrupting the vascularization causes disk degeneration. As we shall see later, the degeneration can be forecast from the type of lesion.

The anterior column is also connected throughout by strong ligaments: The anterior longitudinal ligament extends from the basilar part of the occipital bone to the sacrum along the anterior surfaces of the vertebral bodies and of the disks; the posterior longitudinal ligament is inside the vertebral canal on the posterior surfaces of the body of each vertebra. It extends from the anterior margin of the occipital foramen to the sacral canal. It is a very strong ligament and we shall see in what circumstances it can be injured (luxation, severe sprain, tear-drop fractures).

2. Posterior Arches

The ligamenta flava connect the laminae of adjacent vertebrae. They are particularly thick and resistant.

Laterally the interapophyseal ligaments, which reinforce the interarticular capsules, and the intertransverse ligaments are found. Medially there are the inter- and supraspinous ligaments.

Together these ligaments provide an extremely stable connection between the vertebra and provide the spine with a high degree of mechanical resistance.

B. Functional Anatomy

The vertebral column plays a triple role: static and dynamic roles and the provision of protection for the neuromedullary axis. But it also shows the fundamental characteristics of any bone, i.e., solidity and mobility.

I. Static Role

This role is assured by the superposition of the vertebral bodies and intervertebral disks which form the anterior column or support column. Two factors reinforce the stability of this set: on one hand, the existence in the sagittal plane of the curvatures (cervical and lumbar lordosis, thoracic kyphosis) makes the column more resistant. As a matter of fact, engineers have demonstrated that the resistance of a curved column is proportional to the square of the rate of curvature plus one. The other factor reinforcing stability is the preconstraint stage of the intervertebral disk. In the center of the nucleus pulposus there is a positive pressure that tends to oppose itself spontaneously to the axial compression forces so that its rupture point is raised. The nucleus transmits the pressures to the annulus, which allows the set to have some elasticity.

The anterior column is thus perfectly equipped to resist forces which would otherwise result in axial compression whether applied to an erect spine or to a spine in flexion or lateral flexion. The stability and resistance are quite sufficient for and adapted to the erect posture of man. But there is a natural weakness against horizontal forces, whether these are rotation or shearing movements. Fortunately there are bony and ligamentous abutments that limit the amplitude of such movements, thus preventing premature wear of the intervertebral disk. In the cervical segment the bony abutment's provided by the uncinate facets and the vertical obliquity of the articular processes. In the lumbar segment the antirotation locking is natural, the articular facets being oriented so that their rotation centers do not project onto the vertebral body, but behind the posterior arch in the interspinous space. The thoracic segment, however, has no vertebral bony abutment. On the contrary, the orientation of the articular facets is such that the rotation center projects a long way forward of the intervertebral disk. This explains the vulnerability of the spinal segment to mechanisms acting in torsion rotation. The rib cage could be considered as a bony abutment, however. In fact, statistics show that vertebral lesions caused by torsion-rotation affect particularly the lower thoracic spine, e. g., T11, T12, which are at the same level as the floating ribs.

As far as the ligaments are concerned the range of movement is restricted mainly by the intertransverse ligaments and, to a lesser degree, by the interspinous ligament.

This particular vulnerability of the spine to torsion forces helps us to understand why destruction of the posterior osteoligamentous structures leads to a lesion of the vertebral body with major instability.

II. Dynamic Role

This role devolves mainly on the posterior columns constituted by the accumulation, on the left and right, of the posterior articular pillars. Due to the orientation of its articular facets, each vertebral segment is predisposed to a certain type of movement: flexion and extension take place in the lower cervical segment, whereas rotation is assured by the cervico-occipital joint. The thoracic spine allows rotation movements, whereas the lumbar segment, while permitting flexion and extension, assures antirotation locking. The union between the anterior and the posterior pillars of two adjacent vertebrae constitutes the motor segment. This is made up, from front to back, of the intervertebral disk, the intervertebral foramen, the interapophyseal articulations, and finally, the ligamentum flavum and the interspinous ligament. For each level this motor segment is situated in a single plane, which usually corresponds to the intervertebral disk plane. This dynamic function, assured by the particular architecture of the posterior vertebral structures, accounts to a large extent for the vulnerability of these structures to forces acting by distraction, such as brisk hyperflexion. Involvement of this motor segment in isolation has two major consequences: disk, instability and neurologic damage. Such lesions cause destruction of the ligaments and consequently marked initial or secondary displacements. When the bony vertebral canal is not involved the medulla is exposed either to compression or to section. This is the case, for example, with pure luxations.

III. Neuroprotective Role

At each level the medulla is protected by the vertebral canal constituted, from front to back, by the posterior aspect of the vertebral body, the pedicles, the articular pillars, and the laminae. From the biomechanical point of view the main element of the bony protection is the posterior corporeal aspect situated between the pedicles, or posterior wall. As discussed above, the integrity of the intermedian element is not always desirable in traumatology. Its involvement most often affects the means of union between anterior and posterior pillars (pedicles and laminae) and leads to enlarge-ment of the canal diameters, so that the medulla is spared in case of minor displacements. In contrast, involvement of the posterior wall causes neurologic damage in most cases. The intervertebral foramina, which form a real transverse canal, afford lateral protection for the emergence of the radicular sheaths. Involvement of any one of its walls can be the cause of radicular compression and thus of cervicobrachial or intercostal neuralgiae or of sciatica.

Chapter 2   Trauma of the Cervical Spine

A. Radiologic Investigation Techniques

Radiography of the cervical spine, especially the injured cervical spine, is considered a thankless task, and the radiologist has mostly left it to the technicians. However, it is in fact a medical act that often implicates major responsibility. The radiologist's role in this matter is prominent, involving the selection and conduct of the radiologic investigations on the basis of the clinical signs and/or the degree of urgency.

In the case of polytraumatized patients, i.e., those with impairment of at least two vital functions, it is necessary to determine which procedures have the highest priority. Radiologic investigations should be weighed up against this priority without delaying treatment.

There are some general rules which should be known and taken into account by those who want to perform an accurate and noninvasive investigation on an injured spine:

No patient with an injured spine should be moved until the radiographs have shown that this is safe. Therefore it is necessary to have equipment allowing the different projections to be taken without moving the patient. The radiographs taken in this way are of course poor in quality and unsuitable for semiologic iconography, but their purpose is not to provide precise visualization of the lesions but rather to answer the initial question as to whether the patient can be mobilized. The first-step examination is usually limited to a frontal and a lateral projection. It can be interrupted if it shows evidence of a lesion necessitating an emergency procedure (e.g., cervical luxation) and resumed once this has been reduced.

Large films should be used to obtain visualization of an entire spinal segment. More specific radiographs are only carried out as second-step investigations. For the same reason as an investigation of a diaphysis must include the over- and underlying articulations, an exploration of a spinal segment must show the cranial and the caudal joints. This is particularly true for the cervical and the thoracic segment.

Any unconscious patient — these are usually patients with associated cranial, thoracic and/or abdominal injuries — should have a radiograph taken of the whole spine. This rule is still not widely knwon, and its nonobservance may have dramatic consequences for the patient. One need only think of the nursing care such inconscious patients necessitate and the implications of overlooking a fractured vertebra!

The absence of bone lesions does not allow the conclusion that the discoligamentous structures are not affected. Such lesions are markedly unstable and may rapidly become neurotoxic if they are overlooked. We shall see later what role functional radiography has in the detection of such lesions.

If a vertebral body lesion is diagnosed, involvement of the posterior wall and of the posterior arch must systematically be suspected. Tomographs should then be performed before any treatment is undertaken, unless there is an emergency such as luxation or extradural spinal hematoma.

Finally, it should be kept in mind that there are no inadequate projections as far as traumatic radiology is concerned. Useful information concerning the displacements can be obtained from standard projections. Fracture lines, however, are only visualized when they are parallel to the incident beam.

I. Conventional Roentgenograms

1. Cervico-occipital Joint

a) Frontal Projections

Anteroposterior radiograph through the open mouth, care being taken not to flex the head on the chin, but to tilt the central beam. As a matter of fact, flexion is contraindicated in case of ruptured transverse ligament and in certain types of fracture of the odontoid process.

Method of PELISSIER and OTTONELLI. The patient is told to alternatively open and close his mouth while the roentgenogram is taken: extension of the exposure time by means of a reduction in intensity combined with reduction of the focus-film distance to 60 cm, results in blurring of the lower jawbone so that the two first cervical vertebrae are well displayed.

Frontal projection with intrabuccal anode. The Siemens "dentus" apparatus used for dental and maxillary radiographs allows a magnified frontal projection of the cervico-occipital joint, if the correct procedure is followed. With the patient in a dorsal position, a 24/30 cassette is pushed under the neck and occiput. The intrabuccal anode with a parabolic beam is directed toward the posterior occipital edge. The image obtained in this way is magnified and cleared of the superimposed anterior structures of the face (upper maxillary).

CLARK's transorbital projection. The patient's head is upright with REID's line perpendicular to the film plane. The central beam is directed between the orbitae, and the head is tilted laterally until the central beam falls onto the center of the eye. This projection permits visualization of the occipito-atlantal articulation.

BLONDEAU's and WATER's projections. These provide correct visualization of the odontoid process.

b) Lateral Projections

Strictly lateral projections. These allow recognition of fracture displacements but do not show minor lesions because of the too-perfect superimposition of the lateral structures.

Semioblique lateral projections, with the central beam directed onto the skull or on to C7. These make it possible to avoid superimposition of the lateral structures and thus to visualize unilateral lesions (Fig. 1).

2. Middle and Lower Cervical Spine

In a purposely didactic view, we distinguish three types of investigations, each of which permits a segmental exploration i.e., examination of the vertebral body, of the posterior arch, and of the discoligamentous structures.

a) Vertebral Body

Two projections are usually sufficient, frontal and lateral.

For the frontal view of the body the patient is supine and the central beam is inclined by 15–20° in the podocranial direction. Usually this position straightens the lordosis of the cervical segment, so that a vertical central beam is generally sufficient. With this projection the disks are well displayed, the vertebral plates are parallel, and the uncal facets are individualized. These criteria should always be fulfilled. In case failure, we usually perform this projection a second time after having

taken a lateral projection, first adjusting the central beam to give the best inclination possible.

For the lateral view of the body the patient remains in the supine position. The horizontal central beam is centered onto C4. In the case of torticollis or of scoliotic deviation, the cervical segment must be approached in its concavity. The C7–T1 disk space must be well delineated. There are several ways of achieving this, including pulling on the patient's arms during radiography and auto-traction by the patient by means of straps fixed around the wrists and passing under the patient's feet; the knees are initially flexed at 30°, but the patient is told to slowly stretch out both legs, which produces lowering of the shoulders.

These two projections are quite sufficient for study of the vertebral bodies, the uncal articulations of the posterior wall, and the prevertebral soft tissues.

b) Posterior Arch

α) Pedicles

The best projection is the oblique projection: it delineates the intervertebral foramina.

β) Articular Processes

For the *frontal view* DORLAND's projection is used. The patient is in the supine position; the central beam in craniopodal direction, forming a variable angle for each vertebra depending on the inclination of the posterior articular interspaces relative to the horizontal as seen on the lateral projection. The chin is slightly turned toward the opposite side to that being X-rayed. This projection clearly reveals the superior, inferior, internal, and external margins of the articular processes.

For the *lateral view* (semioblique lateral projection or lateral view of the articular processes) the patient is also supine, and the central beam is inclined by ± 10° to ± 15° relative to the horizontal line. This projection permits visualization of the left and right articular facets: one remains in projection of the cervical canal and is thus correctly visualized, whereas the other is superimposed onto the vertebral body. This projection is especially suitable for the study of the articular facets.

The standard lateral projection or lateral view of the vertebral body does not allow study of the fractures but does permit analysis of their conse-

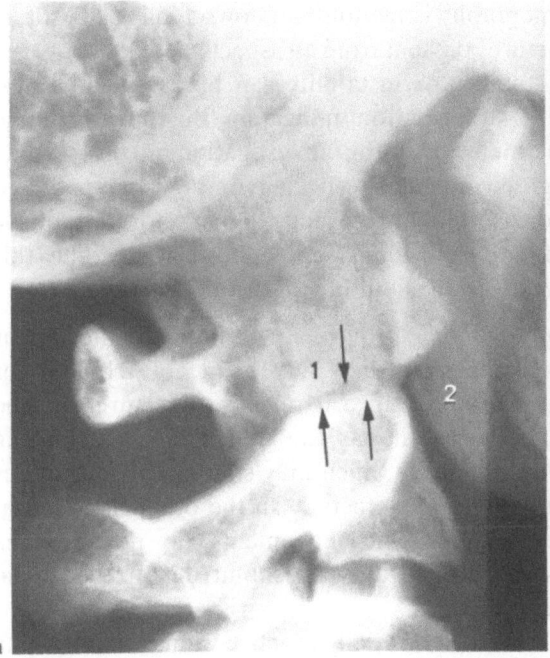 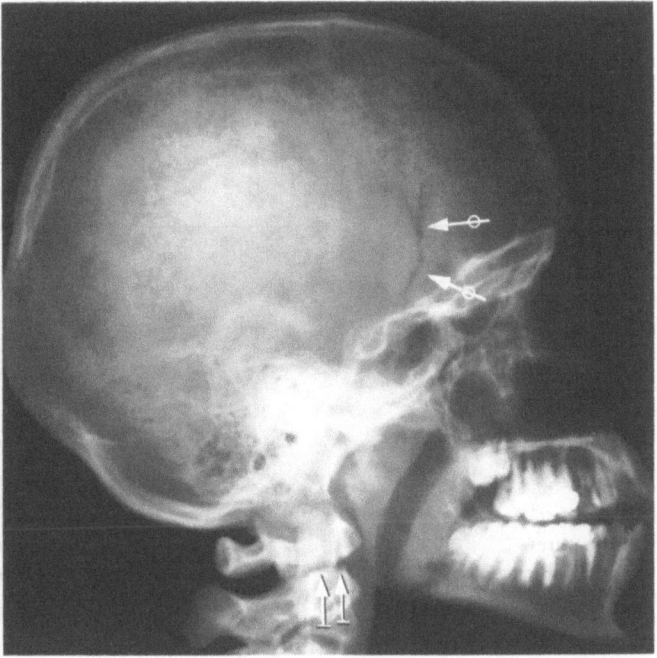

Fig. 1a, b. Fracture of the odontoid process: Role of the incidence. **a** Lateral view of the cervico-occipital joint showing double image of the posterior margins of the lateral masses of the atlas. The fracture line or Mach bands? *(1)* are indicated by *arrows;* swelling of the soft parts of the cavum *(2)* is also visible.

b Lateral radiograph of the skull, showing fracture-dislocation of the odontoid base revealed by a slight rotation of the head with reference to the spine (⊢→), and a frontotemporal fracture (↔)

quences, i.e., displacements. As we shall see later, it is this projection that draws attention to fractures of the articular processes.

In our opinion the *oblique projection* is almost useless for the study of the articular processes, unless it is associated with a craniopodal double obliquity according to DORLAND's technique.

γ) *Laminae*

On a *frontal view* of the body the laminae are projected onto the center of the vertebral body. On a *lateral view* they form the spinolamellar space. The *oblique projection* provides a true frontal view of the lamina and is therefore the one most often used in searching for laminar fractures.

δ) *Spinous and Transverse Processes*

The frontal and lateral views of the vertebral bodies permit correct analysis of the spinous processes.

This analytic study of the projections allows the radiologist to state whether or not a bone lesion is present. Conventional tomograms are then used

for a more detailed study of the extent of the lesions. Tomograms should no longer be used to reveal fractures, but rather to show their extent. For this investigation the same rules should be applied as for the cervico-occipital hinge. In case of complex fractures the investigation will consist of a frontal and a sagittal study. In the case of the presence of parcellar fractures, the projection selected depends on the structure to be X-rayed. For the vertebral body frontal and lateral views are required, for pedicles and laminae, an oblique projection, and for the articular processes, a lateral view (Table 1).

One golden rule should always be respected: the area to be X-rayed must be strictly parallel to the film plane: otherwise the lesions will be strongly minimized.

c) Discoligamentous Structures

The association of an electively painful point, e.g., an interspinous point, and bone integrity or a minor corporeal lesion should automatically suggest involvement of the ligaments. This should be

Table 1. Correlation between radiological incidences and visualization of the anatomic structures

	Standard Frontal view	Dorland's projection	Standard Lateral view	Semioblique projection	Oblique projection	Dynamic studies
Body	+		+			
Pedicle	+				++	
Articular processes		++	+	+++		
Lamina	+		++		++	
Spinous process	+		+			
Disco-ligamentous structures						+++

looked for by means of functional studies performed with following precautions:

Active mobilization with the patient's collaboration. Never force: the pain will serve as a guide for the amplitude of the movements to be made.

Never take dynamic radiographs in unconscious patients including those under a general anesthetic.

Do not have recourse to midsagittal tomographs, but rely rather with standard radiograms.

Avoid performing dynamic studies when discoligamentous lesions seem to exist or when the type of bone lesion, e.g., a tear-drop fracture, suggests the presence of a major discoligamentous instability.

When should the functional investigation be undertaken? In our opinion it can be carried out as soon as the first day, provided the precautions listed above are observed. As a matter of fact, the amplitude of the movements causing discoligamentous lesions could not be intentionally reproduced. This investigation should be carried out at regular intervals so that the point at which an apparently radiologically benign sprain becomes a severe sprain is not overlooked.

II. Tomographic Investigation

Even if the standard investigation has been very carefully carried out, tomograms are indispensable for a precise analysis of the lesions. The role of tomography is twofold: it allows a full review of all fractures present from all aspects so that the degree of stability or instability can be assessed; it also yields information indicating the most suitable treatment. But this investigation involves some degree of danger, especially in high-risk patients, and is often unpleasant for para- or tetraplegic patients. We shall see later at what time this investigation should be performed.

Tomographic Movement. Although the linear movement is the movement of choice for traumatology, since it reveals a fracture line the most clearly, it has the drawback of producing "Mach bands," which may simulate fracture lines (radiological artefacts). On the other hand, complex tomographic movements do not produce linear artifacts but cause blurring of the actual fracture edges.

In fact, in our daily practice we use tomography with complex movement but we regret not being able to vary the section angle, this being dictated by the apparatus.

Positioning of the Patient. Positioning of the patient is the radiologist's task. It must be careful and rigorous, with the patient in a comfortable position allowing a more or less prolonged investigation without decentering, and the clinical criteria for positioning should be respected as scrupulously as possible.

Frontal Tomography. For the cervical spine we take the intervestibular line of WACKENHEIM as a landmark and we avoid flexion.

Lateral Tomography. Anteriorly the nasion, the tip of the chin, and the sternal angle must be in the same plane; posteriorly the external occipital protuberance and the alignement of the spinous processes. When changing the position from frontal to lateral care must be taken not to cause a shearing movement. The patient must be completely immobilized, especially if neurologic signs (cervicobrachial neuralgiae, paraplegia, acute cordonal pain) are present.

Size of the Films. A tomographic investigation should never be focused on a single vertebra. We use large films (24/30 × 2 or 30/40 × 2). To our great surprise this has often allowed us to detect other lesions at various distances from the initial fracture focus that have been overlooked on standard projections.

B. Correlations Between Incidence and Radiographic Image

Our aim is to study the different anterior posterior and lateral vertebral components, or more specifically their radiographic projection, according to CHAUSSÉ's motion procedure, starting from the lateral projection and ending with the frontal projection. The radiographs have been taken at from 5° to 5° on an erect spine, as is most often the case with patients with cervical traumas who are examined in the supine position. In the light of the results we distinguish four rotation sectors that have a global amplitude of 20°, i. e., 5–20°, 25–40°, 45–60°, and 65–80°. The 0° incidence corresponds to the lateral and 90° to the frontal view.

First Rotation Sector (5–20°). In this sector there is no superimposition of the posterior articular columns. The articular interspaces can be easily identified. At a 20° rotation the posterior articular columns are perfectly visualized. One projects in the cervical canal and the other is partly superimposed on the vertebral body. This is the incidence of choice for detecting luxations and unilateral fractures of the articular pillars and articular processes (Fig. 2).

Moreover, simultaneously we can see the reduction in the apophysolaminar space, and the spreading-out of the homolateral pedicle. At a rotation of about 20–25° the spinolaminar line becomes tangential to the homolateral posterior interarticular line.

Second Rotation Sector (25–40°). The pedicle is increasingly stretched. The posterior articular interlines can no longer be identified. The laminae project themselves onto the articular pillars. They are tangential to their posterior aspect at 25° and to their anterior aspect at 40–45°, and project into their center at 35–40° (Fig. 3).

This is the incidence of choice for detection of transverse fractures of the laminae and display of the posterior connections of the nerve roots with the foramen intervertebrale. Note that at 30–35°

the contralateral pedicle is seen as a cockade-like image in the center of the vertebral body.

Third Rotation Sector (45–60°). At 45° the so-called anterior or posterior oblique standard projection is taken. The intervertebral foramen is seen with its largest projection area and is free from any superimposition. The pedicle is maximally spread and we can distinguish its connections with the uncal facets (Fig. 4).

Beyond 55° the spinous process projects itself in the intervertebral foramen. This rotation field permits a good analysis of the pediculocorporeal junction.

Fourth Rotation Sector (65–80°). This sector is undoubtedly the one that yields the least information. However, it permits quite a detailed study of the uncovertebral articulations (Fig. 5).

This summary shows that the variations are homogeneous and homothetic for each vertebral level. Therefore we can see a vertical and parallel alignment of the different radiologic lines, i. e.,

Alignment of the anterior corporeal aspects (anterior wall) or of the posterior corporeal aspects (posterior wall)

Alignment of the anterior and posterior aspects of the articular pillars

Alignment of the spinolaminar lines

Alignment of the spinous processes

This investigation has been carried out on an erect spine. It would have provided almost similar results with a lordotic cervical segment, but instead of being rectilinear the lines would be curved, though still parallel.

A brisk segmental disalignment involving a single vertebral level should suggest a unilateral lesion of the posterior arch. This general rule has often permitted us to detect a fracture or a unilateral luxation by means of an appropriate tomographic investigation in difficult cases.

Figure 6 illustrates an experimental unilateral luxation of dried bone. The radiologic findings entirely confirm the signs we had found in vivo, i. e., the indirect signs of lateralized antelisthesis syndrome: moderate antelisthesis on the lateral radiogram (disalignment of the posterior wall), being more pronounced on the side of the lesion and less so on the opposite on the oblique view;

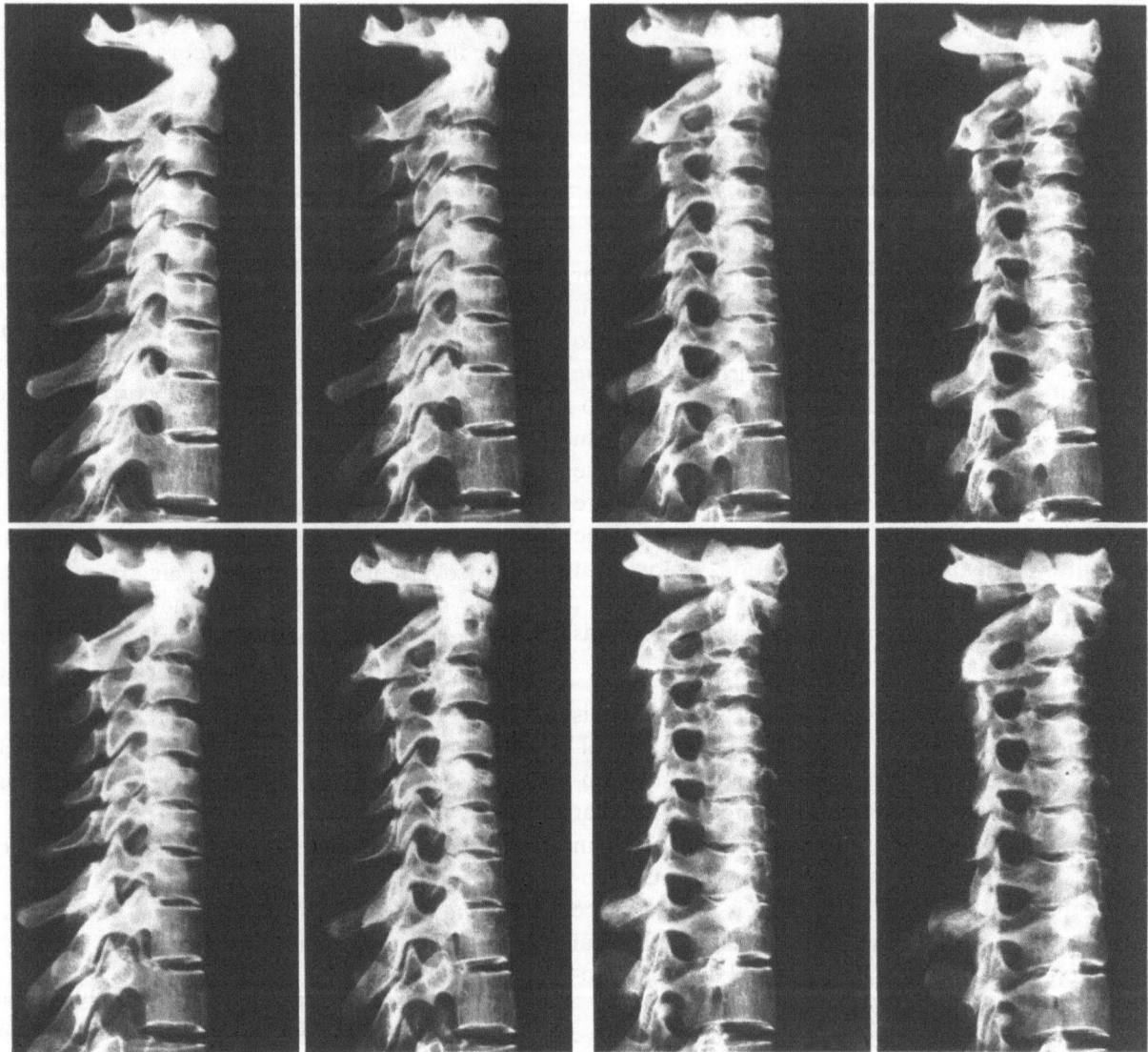

Fig. 2. Radiographic image of the spine in the first rotation sector (5–20°) $\frac{5|10}{15|20}$

Fig. 3. Radiographic image of the spine in the second rotation sector (25–40°) $\frac{25|30}{35|40}$

slight disalignment of the spinous process, moving to the side of the luxation; widening of the intervertebral foramen; and abnormal uncovertebral interspace.

Lateroflexion and rotation have little influence on the lower cervical spine, these movements having a limited amplitude and always being conjugate. They produce disalignment of the vertebral elements in the horizontal direction. This is very frequent in torticollis, and easily recognized on the frontal projection. On the lateral projection, however, there is no vertical superimposition of the right and left lateral parts of the arches, which means that visualization of the posterior articular interspaces and of the disk space is poor, but the vertical alignment of the lines described above is preserved.

C. Guide for Interpretation

The first radiographic picture must be analysed with the most extreme preciseness. The more so

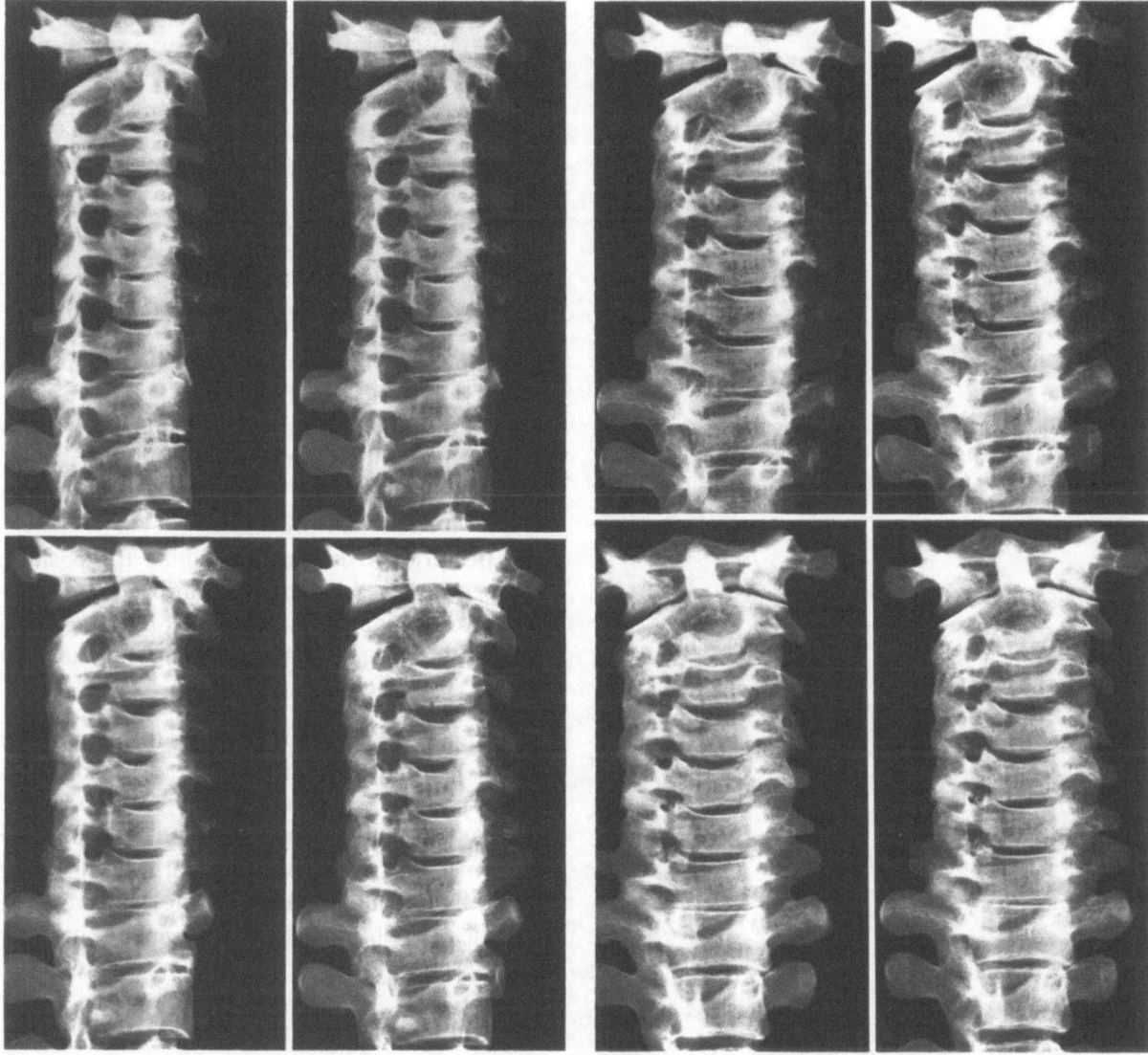

Fig. 4. Radiographic image of the spine in the third rotation sector (45–60°) $\frac{45|50}{55|60}$

Fig. 5. Radiographic image of the spine in the fourth rotation sector (65–80°) $\frac{65|70}{75|80}$

that these first documents are most often the first-step radiographs or so-called necessity projections. Under these conditions the radiologist has no semiological reference data. He must be able to recognize the various vertebral structures whatever projection has been utilized to take the pictures. It is most important to diagnose the lesions and the displacements of the posterior arches, since these are the most neurotoxic lesions. Therefor we would like to propose an interpretation guide based on a vertical and horizontal reference lines.

I. Cervico-occipital Joint

The reference points on the cervico-occipital joint are well known, we shall therefore only enumerate them.

On the frontal projection there are from top to bottom:

WACKENHEIM's intervestibular line
FISCHGOLD and METZGER's bidigastric line
The bimastoid line

The mediatrixes of theses three lines are super-

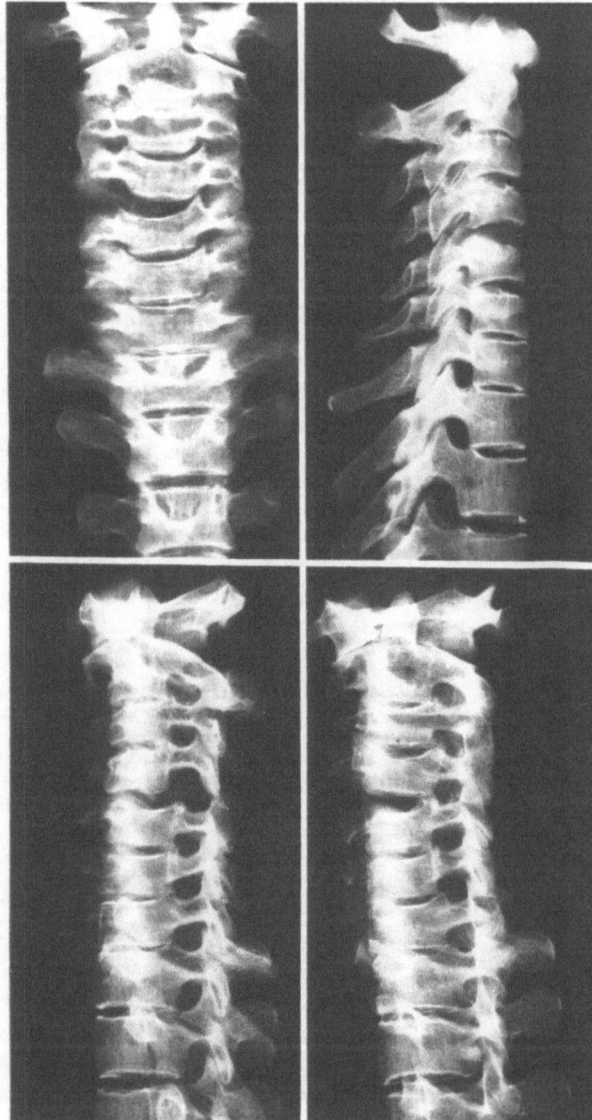

Fig. 6. Experimental unilateral luxation of dried bone

imposed and pass through the symmetry axe of odontoid process. The lateral masses of the atlas and of the axis are symmetrical in shape, size and configuration with regard to these mediatrixes.

On the lateral projection we shall retain:

    CHAMBERLAIN's and/or McGREGOR's palato-occipital line

    WACKENHEIM, VROUSOS and THIEBAUT's basilar line

These two lines cross each other Theoretically at the level of the postero-superior aspect of the odontoid process.

Any shifting of the odontoid process with regard to this cross-point must lead to suspect a cervico-occipital joint lesion.

II. Mobile Cervical Segment from C3 to C7

1. Alignment of the Vertebrae

In the lateral view the study comprises analysis of the following lines from front to back (Fig. 7):

The anterior wall, formed by the alignment of the anterior aspects of the vertebral bodies

The posterior wall, formed by the alignment of the posterior aspects of the vertebral bodies

The anterior articular line joining the tips of the superior articular processes

The posterior articular line joining the posterior aspects of the inferior articular processes

The spinolaminar lines, formed at the junction on the midline by the insertion of the laminae on the spinous processes.

We may add to these bony lines the prevertebral soft tissue line, which is essential for the detection of prespinal hematomas.

The study of these lines shows that we now have three median criteria (the anterior wall, the posterior wall, and the spinolaminar line) and two lateral criteria (the anterior articular line and the posterior articular line).

In Chap. 2, Sect. B, we saw that on the straight spine these different lines remain parallel to each other whatever the incidence of the beam when the projection is orthogonal: the lines converge or diverge when the projection is oblique.

On a frontal view the following lines are seen in the following order:

Alignment of the spinous processes

Alignment of the pedicles

Alignment of the external aspects of the articular processes or external articular line

We thus have one posterior median criterion (alignment of the spinous processes) and two anterolateral criteria (the alignment of the pedicles and the external articular lines).

The combined interpretation of these frontal and lateral lines allows recognition of nine sectors, represented on the schematic of Fig. 8.

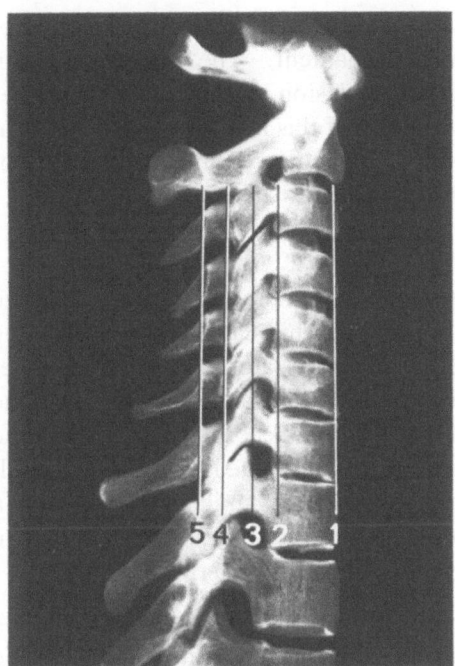

Fig. 7. Lateral view of the mobile cervical segment of the spine

The lesions in each sector involve a particular toxicity, i. e.,

Medullotoxicity for lesions of the central axis (2–5)

Radiculotoxicity for the lesions of the median external sector (4–6)

Vasculotoxicity for the lesions of the anterolateral sector (1–3)

2. Distances Between the Vertebrae

At each level this study consists in analysis of the relationships between the homologous structures of two adjacent vertebrae, i. e.,

Distance between the pedicles (frontal view).

Distance between the spinous processes on the frontal view; on the lateral view this distance is measured at the level of the apophysolaminar junction.

Posterior interapophyseal articular interspaces (lateral view).

Uncovertebral interspaces (frontal and oblique views).

Size of the intervertebral foramina (oblique view).

In normal cases these relationships are identical on the left and on the right and variations harmonize from one vertebral level to the other. Any sudden localized change in these relationships must suggest the existence of a uni- or bilateral lesion.

D. Basic Radiosemiology of Cervical Lesions

I. Upper Cervical Segment C0 to C2

1. Lesions of the Atlas Vertebra

Lesions of the atlas, excepting those involving the transverse ligaments, are usually benign. Any toxicity is due to associated luxation. Fractures of the posterior and anterior arches are easily diagnosed, but those of the lateral masses may be more difficult to detect and are often only visible on tomograms.

Isolated fractures of the posterior arch are seen as linear translucencies easily visible on slightly oblique projections. There is usually no displacement, since the posterior arch is attached to the occiput and to the axis by strong musculoligamentous structures. Usually the fracture line is located at the site of lesser resistance, just behind the lateral masses. Exceptionally it may be located on the midline and must then be distinguished from a posterior rachischisis.

Isolated fracture of the anterior arch is uncommon, but it is often seen in association with other vertebral lesions. When bilateral it is responsible for anterior atlanto-odontoid diastasis, which must be differentiated from transverse ligament involvement.

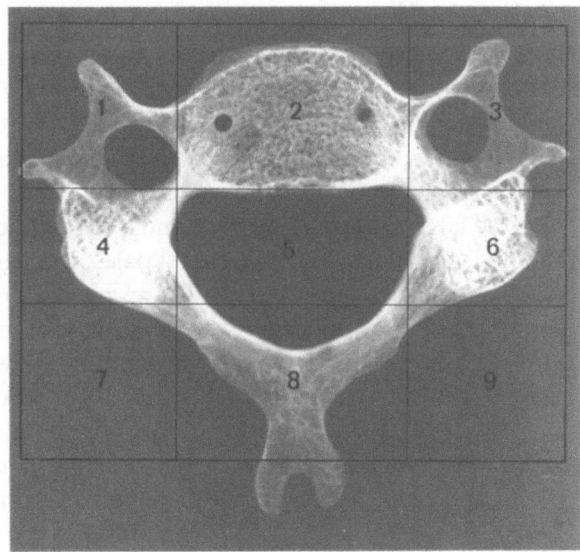

Fig. 8. Schematic showing the lines seen in the axial view determining the toxicity diagram

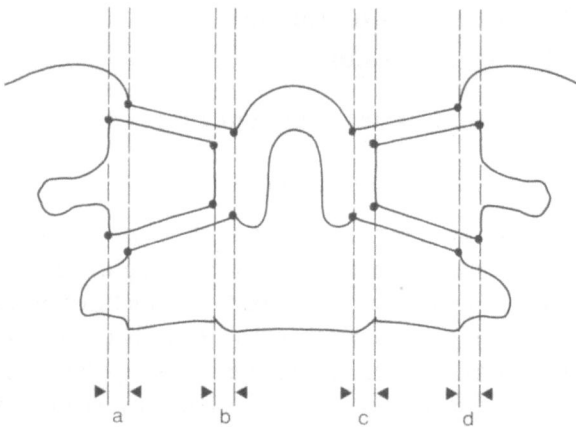

Fig. 9. JEFFERSON'S fracture: schematic representation on the frontal view

a) Fractures of the Lateral Masses

The unilateral and more fraquent bilateral fractures of the lateral masses of the atlas are divided into two main groups: fracture dislocation with intact lateral masses and fracture of the lateral masses proper.

In both cases the cause of injury is a compression mechanism in which the traumatic force is perpendicular to the vertex. The lateral masses are compressed between the occipital condyles and the axis body, and they tend to be displaced away from the midline. This displacement is facilitated by their anatomical predisposition.

α) Fracture-Dislocation

A frontal transbuccal view shows a bilateral lateral offset of the lateral masses with normal occipitoatlantal and atlantoaxial interspaces, associated with gaping of the atlantodental space. On each side the gaping is usually equal to the offset (Fig. 9). In this case the lateral masses are intact, and fracture lines should be looked for in the weakest parts, i. e., the anterior and posterior arches. There are at least three fracture foci, usually two posterior and one anterior one. They are visible on a lateral view. Due to the transverse dislocation involvement of the transverse ligament, stretching or rupture, may occur, which can be evidenced by anterior odontoatlantal gaping seen on the dynamic study in flexion.

Such a lesion is only slightly neurotoxic, since it increases the cervical canal diameter in all direc-

tions: it depends on the degree of involvement of the transverse ligament. The absence of an osteocartilaginous lesion of the lateral masses allows assimilation of this involvement to subluxations or lateral dislocations, which usually do not induce arthritic changes.

β) Fracture Proper

This fracture is due to the same mechanism as the previous type but in this case, instead of being laterally subluxated, the lateral mass exploses between the occipital condyle and the axis body. The radiologic image differs according as whether the orientation of the fracture line is sagittal or frontal. This type of lesion is usually unilateral; it is due to a vertical compression force acting on the spine while it is not straight but inclined to the side.

Anteroposteriorly Directed Fractures (Fig. 10). A frontal transbuccal view shows on the injured side the lateral offset of one lateral mass and narrowing of the odontoatlantal distance, and on the opposite side good visualization of the condyloatlantal and atlantoaxial interspaces, with a normal condyloaxial distance. These lesions are usually not visible on a lateral view.

Transversally Directed Fractures (Fig. 11). On a frontal view the following radiologic signs attract attention:

The lateral mass overlaps onto the occipital condyle and the body of the axis; the occipitoatlantal and atlantoaxial interspaces are poorly visible or

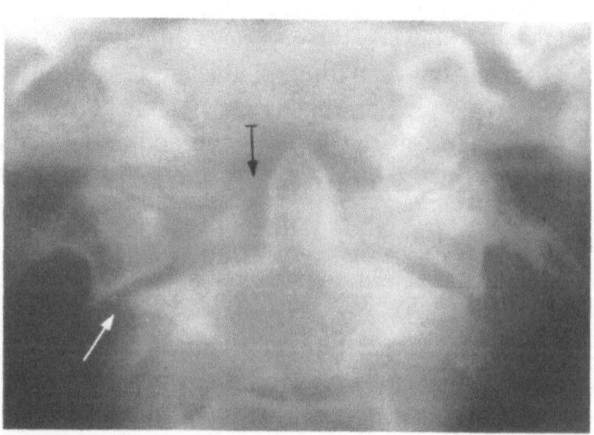

Fig. 10. Fracture of the right lateral mass of the atlas, with lateral offset (→) and narrowing of the odontoatlantal distance (↦)

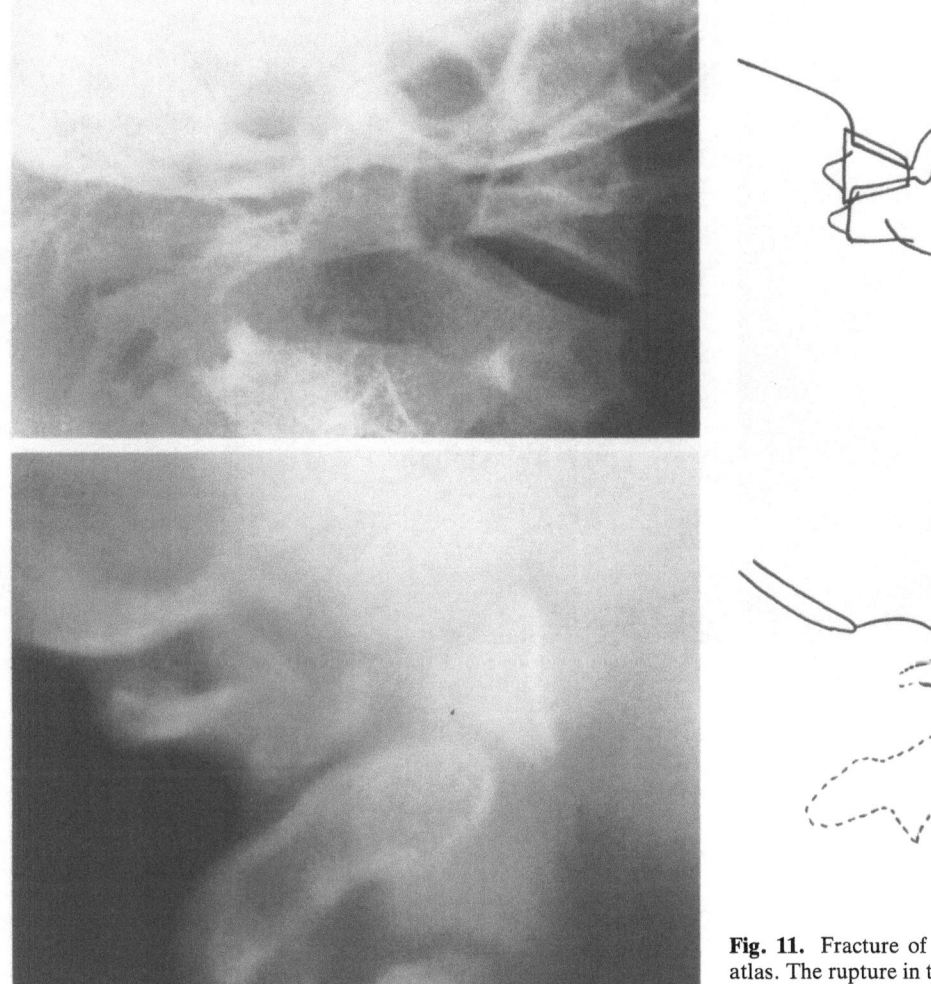

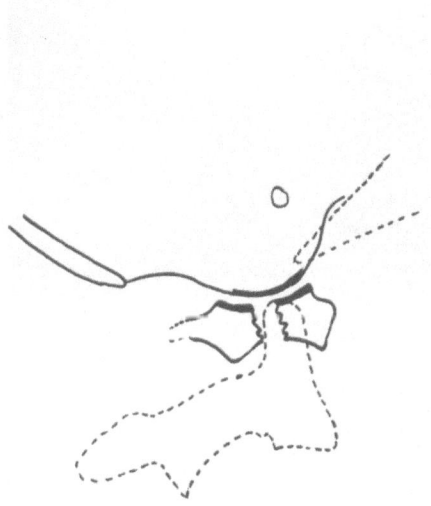

Fig. 11. Fracture of the right lateral mass of the atlas. The rupture in the continuity has a transverse direction

even absent; the condyloaxial height is diminished; and the injured lateral mass has convex medial and lateral aspects.

More information is gained from the lateral view, which shows shifting or duplication of the posterior aspect of the lateral masses, and above all, from the lateral tomogram, which gives the best visualization of the following bone lesions: interfragmental diastasis with anterior and/or posterior offset of the lateral masses relative to the occipital condyle and to the axis body.

Unfortunately the radiologic images are not always so typical; it may then be necessary to look for minor and more localized lesions. There could, for instance, be a parcellar fracture of a superior or inferior lateral angle or of a medial margin caused

by a bone fragment detached from the lateral mass due to the action of the transverse ligament via its tubercle.

Like anteroposterior fractures, this type of fracture is only slightly medullotoxic, but it has a poorer prognosis since it can lead to atlantoaxial arthrosis and thus to restricted rotation, and also to ARNOLD's neuralgia.

b) Luxations and Subluxations

These lesions are seldom found in isolation, being mostly associated with other fractures and therefore often missed. They usually occur in the course of violent traumas or polytraumas. In severe traumas to the spine in children they are most often seen at the level of the cervico-occipital joint.

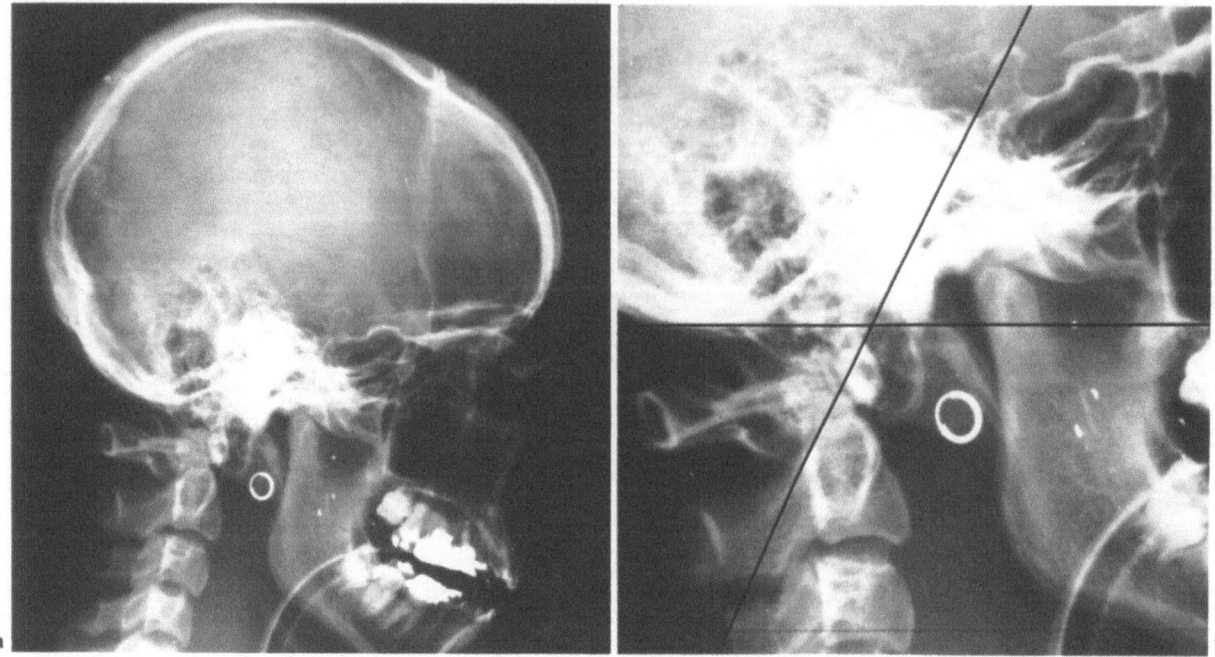

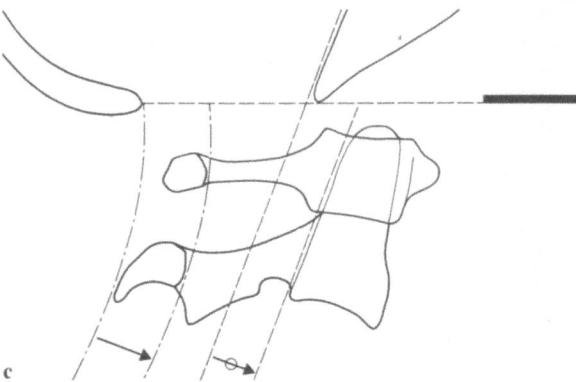

Fig. 12 a–c. Atlanto occipital luxation. **a, b** Traumatic anterior atlanto occipital luxation. **c** Traumatic posterior atlanto occipital luxation: Schematic representation. Contrarily to anterior luxation (**a b**) we note an anterior shiftinf of the spinolaminar line (–·–) and also an anterior displacement (⟷) of the dens, witch is no longer at a tangent to WACKENHEIM-VROUSOS-THIEBAUT's line

Diagnosis is difficult and requires of the reference lines and knowledge of the limits of normality depending on the utilized incidence and on the degree of mobility of the cervical spine with regard to the skull base.

α) Occipitoatlantal Luxation

Occipitoatlantal luxations (Fig. 12) are very rare. Death is inevitable due to involvement of the bulbomedullary junction. In this case the only role of radiology is forensic. However, subluxations without bulbar compression can be diagnosed from radiograms. In the case of anterior subluxation the dens, which is normally at a tangent to the lines of WACKENHEIM, VROUSOS, and THIEBAUT, is displaced backwards. This displacement is accompanied by a significant hematoma of the prevertebral soft parts, so that the oropharyngeal translucency

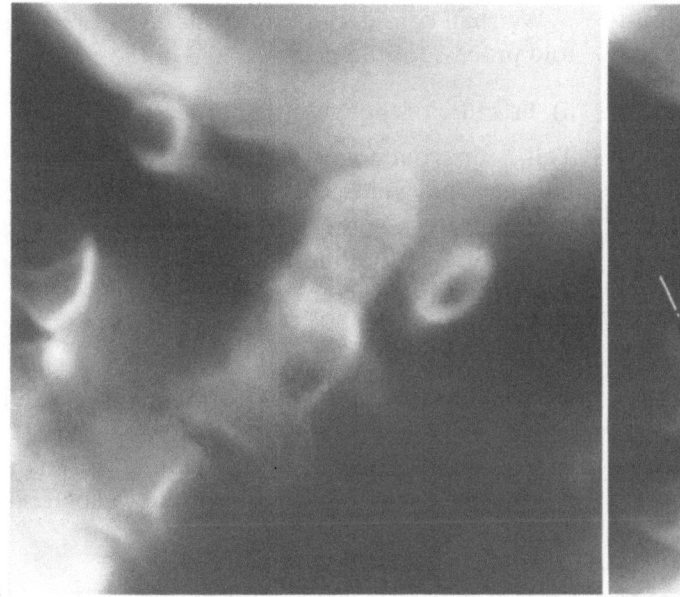 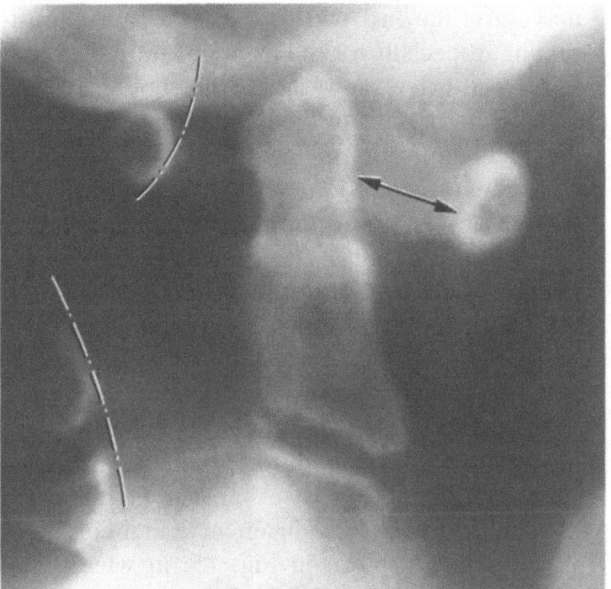

a

b

Fig. 13a, b. Anterior atlantoaxial luxation, frontal view in neutral position (**a**) and in flexion position (**b**). The frontal view in flexion position shows anterior odontoatlantal diastasis (↔) and disalignment of the spinolaminar line (–·–·–)

(the so-called fat line, which corresponds to the retropharyngeal space) is pushed forward. The posterior arch of the atlas is displaced backwards over an equal distance relative to the posterior margin of the foramen magnum, producing the posterior translation of the spinolaminar line.

β) Anterior Odontoatlantal Luxation

The term atlantoaxial luxation (Fig. 13) is used to mean involvement of the transverse ligament. This lesion is caused by a forced hyperflexion movement during which the dens abuts at the posterior surface against the ligament and ruptures it. Such a mechanism can also cause fracture of the odontoid base, in which case the transverse ligament remains intact and displacement is due to involvement of the posterior or anterior longitudinal ligament. The diagnosis is made on a lateral projection taken in flexion. This displays the diastasis between the anterior arch of the atlas and the odontoid process. This distance varies from 2 mm in the adult to 5 mm in children. On account of the magnification factor these figures are of course unreliable. In our daily practice we use different criterion: the anterior odontoatlantal diastasis must be smaller than the normal prevertebral soft parts at the level of C3.

γ) Rotation-Luxation of the Atlas on the Axis

Rotation luxation (Fig. 14) occurs following a trauma in the rotation position. Clinically it causes torticollis. This irreducible pathologic position makes X-raying difficult. Tomograms are often

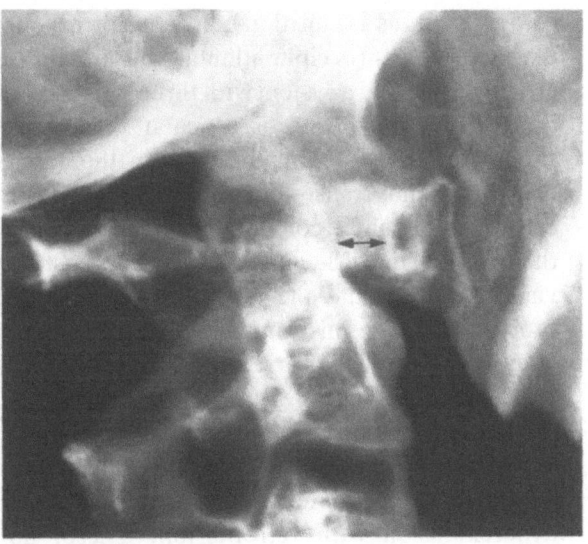

Fig. 14. Rotation-luxation of C1–C2, lateral view. The atlas is viewed obliquely, whereas the axis remains lateral. The anterior arch of the atlas is projected onto a lateral mass. Note the odontoatlantal diastasis showing the involvement of the transverse ligament (lateral position of the rotation pivot) (↔)

necessary; they are carried out after careful positioning, especially for the frontal view.

A frontal view shows lateral offset of one lateral mass with widening of the odontoatlantal distance and medial offset of the contralateral lateral mass with diminished odontolateral distance. These reserve offsets are responsible for the asymmetry of the lateral masses. The spinous process of C2 remains centered on the midline.

A lateral view is more informative, the atlas being visualized obliquely with its anterior arch projected more or less onto a lateral mass.

In fact there are two different types of rotation luxation, and they have different prognoses. In one case the rotation axis passes through the odontoid process, the transverse ligament remaining uninvolved: this is shown in Fig. 15, in which both lateral masses are luxated. In the other case the axis passes through the atlantoaxial articulation, and due to the rupture of the transverse ligament, only one lateral mass is luxated.

Radiologically, the presence of an anterior odontoatlantal diastasis is the sign of a lateralized rotation axis. This type of lesion is neurotoxic.

2. Lesions of the Axis Vertebra

Both functionally and biomechanically, the axis is a transitional vertebra. From the architectural point of view it acts as a transition between a prop system with two pillars (occipitoatlantal and atlantoaxial articulations) and a system with three pillars (vertebral bodies and posterior articular pillars). The single vertebral force at the level of the cervicooccipital joint is transmitted to the subjacent cervical segment by three components: one anterior, via the body and the disk, and the two others posterior, via the pedicle and the posteroinferior articular process. Due to this anatomical disposition the atlantoaxial articulation ensures that almost the full range of rotation movements is possible.

Fractures of the axis are not due to any one single mechanism. The most common causes are certainly hyperflexion movements with antepulsion and hyperextension with retropulsion. These, however, are commonly associated with vertical forces acting either by compression (heavy object hitting the vertex) or by distraction (hanging or brisk deceleration).

We shall consider in turn fractures of the odontoid process, of the pedicles, and of the body.

a) Fracture of the Odontoid Process

This is the commonest fracture and paradoxically the one about which least is known. There are three types: I, affecting the tip of the odontoid process; II, fracture of the body of the odontoid process; and III, basilar fracture of the odontoid process.

α) Fracture of the Tip (Type I)

This is the least common type. The lesion is stable and corresponds to osteoligamentous tearing. It is usually accompanied by other, more severe, spinal lesions and is discovered during the tomographic studies.

β) Fracture of the Neck (Type II)

The horizontal or oblique fracture line runs right through the compact bone, where consolidation is slow and delicate. Because of the antalgic posture of the patient the fracture line is not readily displayed, so that it must often be suspected from indirect signs that are easily visible on lateral roentgenograms. These signs are: swelling of the prevertebral soft tissues; angulation of the anterior aspect of C2; and anterior or posterior displacement of the posterior tubercle of the atlas relative to the spinolaminar line.

The presence of any of these indirect signs associated with complaints of pain in the upper cervical segment must lead to the performance of tomograms. In this case too, the lateral cuts are the most informative. Indeed, frontal tomograms taken with the head in hyperextension (safety position and antalgic posture) could fail to reveal the lesions.

The following signs should be considered:

The fracture line is usually located on either side of a line joining the lower margins of the spinous process and the anterior arch of the atlas.

The fracture line is thin, irregular, and crenellated.

It runs in a horizontal, oblique, sagittal, or frontal direction.

The displacements are conditioned by the orientation of the fracture line and by the involvement of the vertical intra- or extraspinal ligaments. Analysis of these displacements is essential, since it dictates the therapy to be applied.

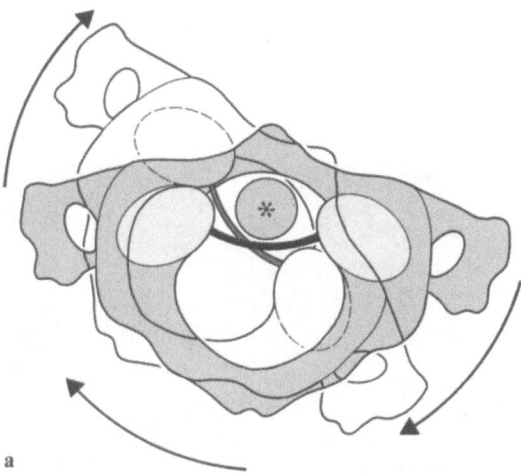

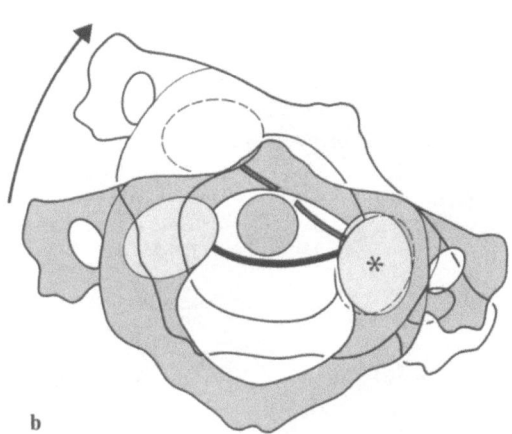

Fig. 15a, b. Rotation-luxation of the atlas the axis. **a** The rotation axis passes through the odontoid process (*). **b** The rotation axis is in lateral position (left articular pillar) (*)

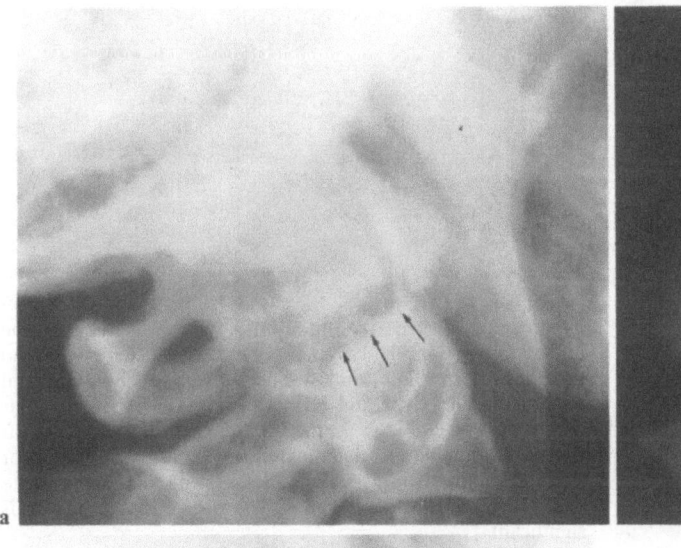

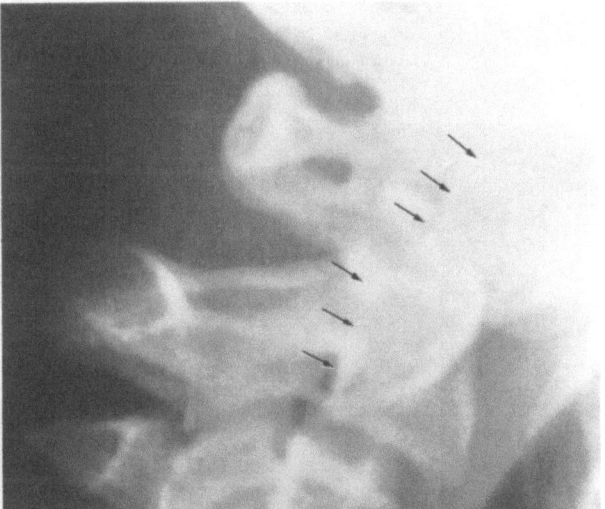

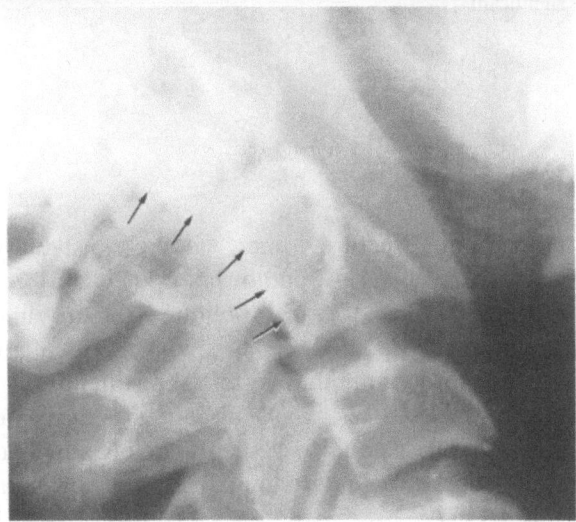

Fig. 16a–c. Fracture of the odontoid neck. Dynamic lateral radiograph of the cervico-occipital joint. The neutral position **(a)** reveals transverse subluxation and a double image of the posterior arches of C1. The flexion **(b)** and extension **(c)** positions show anterior and posterior displacement *(arrows)* (global instability)

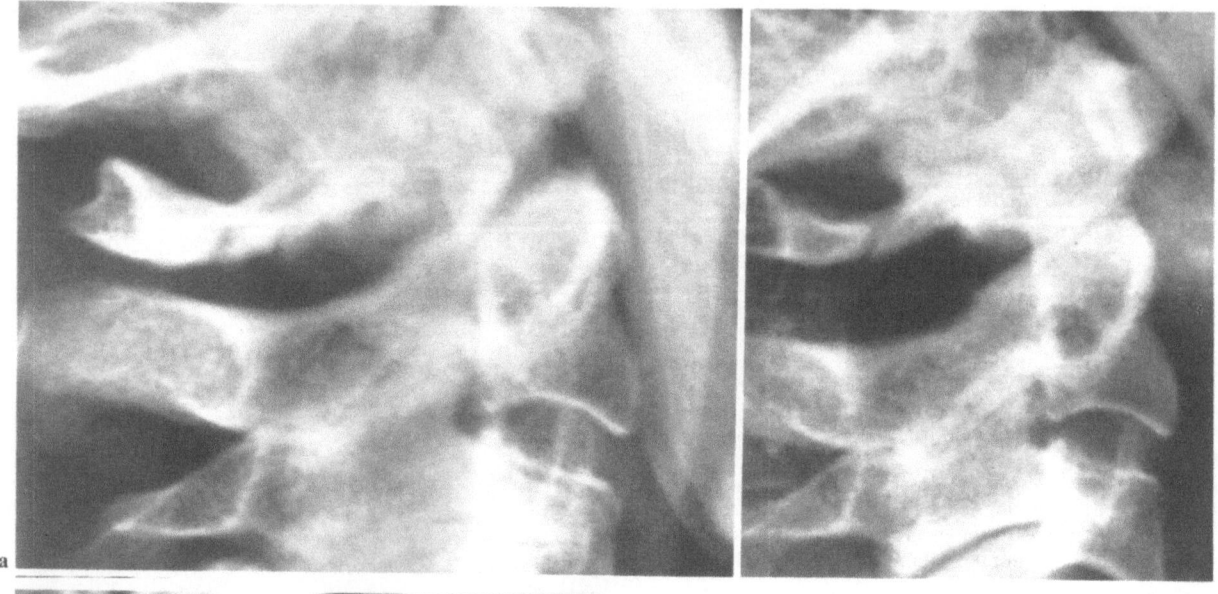

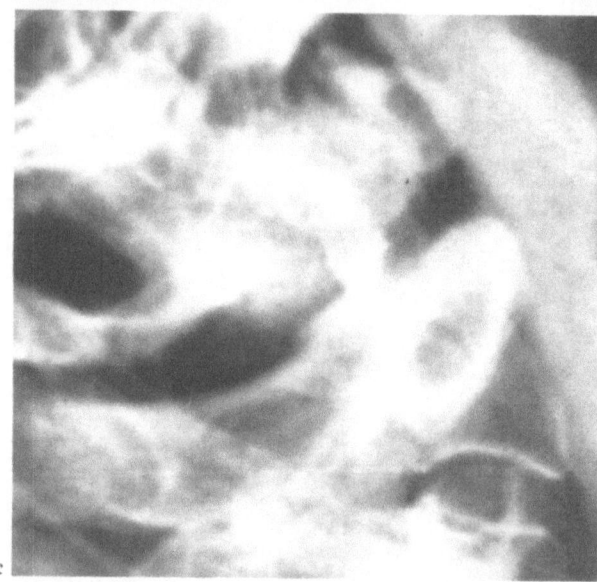

Fig. 17a–c. Fracture of odontoid process resulting from hyperextension. **a** At the initial investigation 2 days after the injury the patient had upper cervicalgiae. There were no neurologic signs. The fracture line runs obliquely down- and backward. The right and left posterior arches of the atlas vertebra are fractured. Note the swelling of the prevertebral soft tissues. **b** Reduction in slight flexion, associated with a posterior graft. **c** Secondary displacement necessitating treatment despite patients use of a Minerva collar. The risk of pseudarthrosis is significant

The instability can be anterior, posterior, lateral, or global. Isolated posterior displacements are the most neurotoxic and require emergency stabilization treatment. They are often responsible for death occurring in a pseudocontext of delirium tremens.

Schematically we might say that the orientation of the fracture lines determines the secondary instability:

Horizontal fracture line: global instability, anterior, posterior, and/or lateral (Fig. 16)

Downward and forward oblique fracture line: anterior instability due to involvement of the posterior longitudinal vertebral ligament

Downward and backward oblique fracture line: Posterior instability due to involvement of the anterior longitudinal vertebral ligament (Fig. 17).

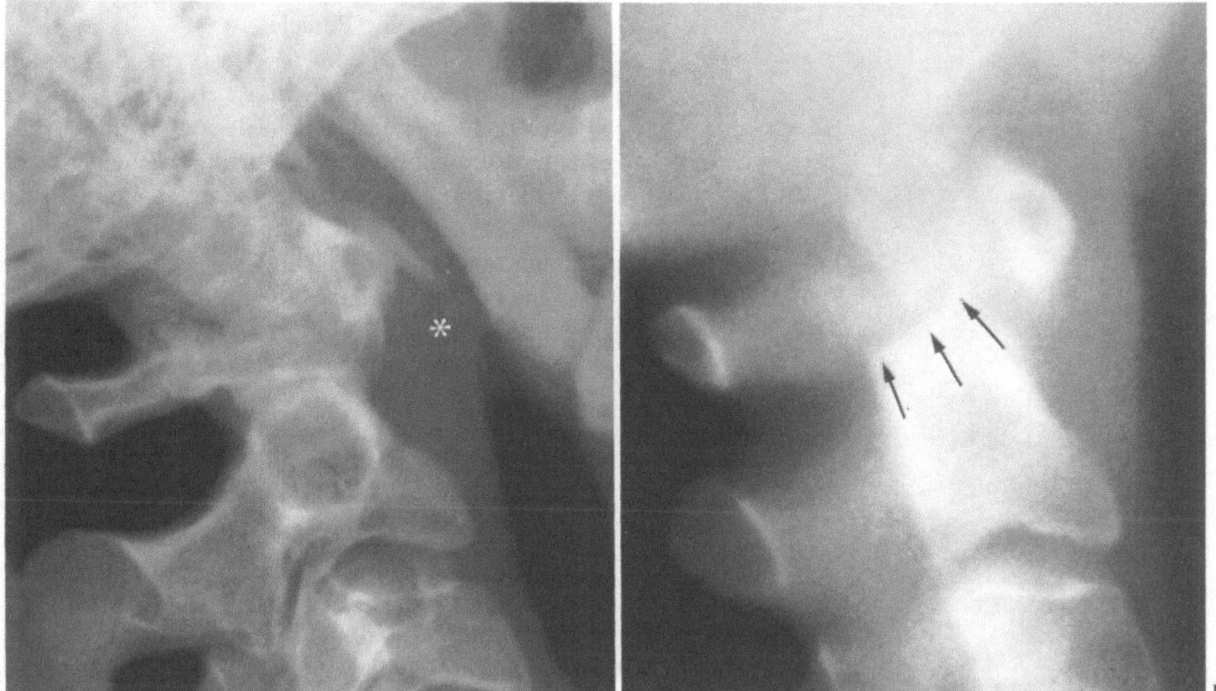

Fig. 18a, b. Mobile pseudarthrosis of an odontoid neck fracture revealed on the occasion of a new trauma. The edges of the fracture are dense and smooth *(arrows)*. The dynamic study in the flexion position reveals an instability. Conventional films X-ray picture **(a)** reveals swelling of the prevertebral soft tissues (∗). The tomogram is also shown **(b)**

The instability should be checked by active dynamic studies carefully carried out in conscious patients. From these studies we decide the orthopedic immobilization modalities (in the reduction position) or the mode of surgical fixation (graft, interspinous wiring, JUDET's first or second mode, screwing).

γ) Basilar Fracture (Type III)

In this type the fracture line is located at the corporeodental junction, within the spongy bone. This junction is a weaker part and corresponds to the embryologic location of the intervertebral atlantoaxial disk. This anatomical predisposition explains why the direction of the fracture line follows that of the former intervertebral disk, downward and forward. The fracture is thus commonly responsible for anterior instability in flexion. In contrast to type II, the fracture of the odontoid base easily undergoes consolidation, even if it has been neglected (Fig. 19).

In some cases the fracture line extends to the axis body and becomes transarticular. This is the classic

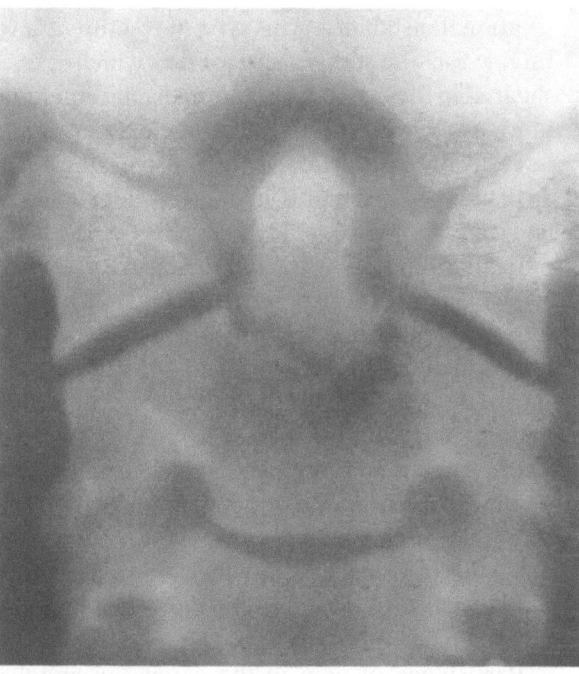

Fig. 19. Fracture of the base of the odontoid, in the spongy bone, sustained in a traffic accident. No neurologic lesions were found. Orthopedic treatment led to consolidation within 3 months

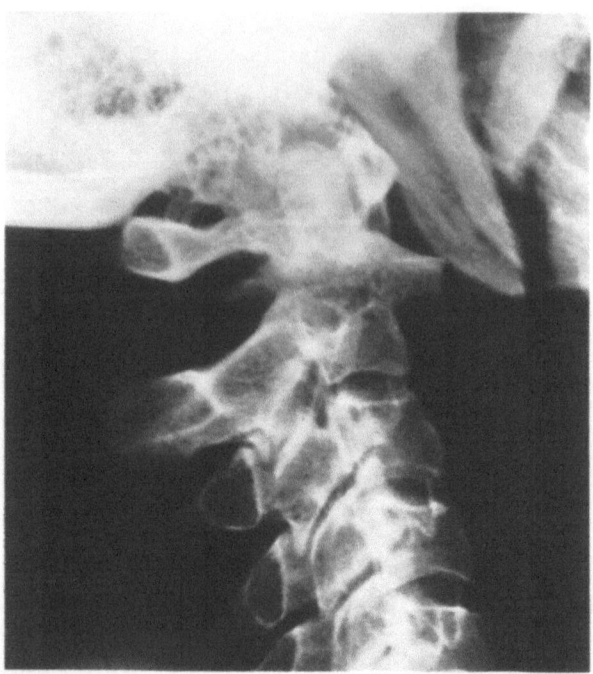

Fig. 20. English policeman's helmet fracture without neurologic damage, due to a road injury. During surgery (internal fixation) an acute subdural hematoma occurred. This lateral projection reveals

"English policeman's helmet fracture (ROY-CAMILLE et al. 1980)." It is characterized by rotational instability. This type of fracture is a real threat for the nerve structures, which can be sheared in the event of a rotation displacement, the more easily when the fracture line extends further laterally onto the articular surface, i. e., the base of an English policeman's helmet is wider (Figs. 20 and 21).

In children basilar fracture leads to epiphysiolysis; we distinguish two varieties (Figs. 22 and 23):

Acute epiphysiolysis, which is usually fatal unless reduction can be carried out immediately after the trauma. Clinically there is flaccid tetraplegia with cardiorespiratory arrest.

Progressive epiphysiolysis, which usually cannot be diagnosed from the initial data for two reasons. The fracture line passes through the vestigial C1/2 disk, the translucency of which normally persists until the age of 4 years. On the other hand, the displacement is progressive.

Persistence of pain in the cervico-occipital region or the occurrence of a torticollis lead to perform control X-rays which then afford the proof of the lesion.

b) Fracture of the Pedicles

Fracture of the pedicles is also called traumatic spondylolysis, or hangman's fracture. In 1913 WOOD JONES described a lesion of the cervical spine following a judicial hanging. He believed that this lesion resulted from hyperextension with violent distraction and destruction of the discoligamentous structures. Death was caused by section of the bulbomedullary junction. Since then, different authors have reported on this lesion occurring in other circumstances, such as traffic accidents, in association with injuries to the face or skull. We must therefore admit, as a second mechanism, the hypothesis of an axial compression force. In contrast to the fractures of the odontoid process, in which even forced flexion extension movements alone can cause the lesions, the indispensable condition for the occurrence of a pedicular fracture is a violent and sudden ascending (distraction) or descending (compression) axial force passing through the force lines of the axis.

Only the direction of this force determines the nature of the discoligamentous lesions and the factors of instability. The fracture is usually bilateral and causes widening of the cervical canal diameter. If death does not occur immediately due to section of the medulla, the prognosis is paradoxically good in spite of the discoligamentous instability responsible for secondary displacements. Usually the roentgenographic diagnosis is easily made on a lateral view. The fracture line presents as a vertical or oblique interruption, extending from the upper margin of the pedicle to the inferior articular facet of C2. This is the pure pedicular fracture. The diastasis between the body and the posterior arch of the axis is almost constant, and becomes more easily visible with increasing severity.

But there are not only pure pedicular fractures, and the fracture line can extend from the superior aspect of the pedicle to the inferior articular process, from which it detaches a fragment that is displaced into the intervertebral foramen (pediculoarticular fracture) or toward the posteroexternal part of the vertebral body (corporeopedicular fracture). In some cases it can be associated with a fracture of the odontoid process.

The radiologic investigation comprises a study of the discoligamentous instability by means of flexion-extension studies.

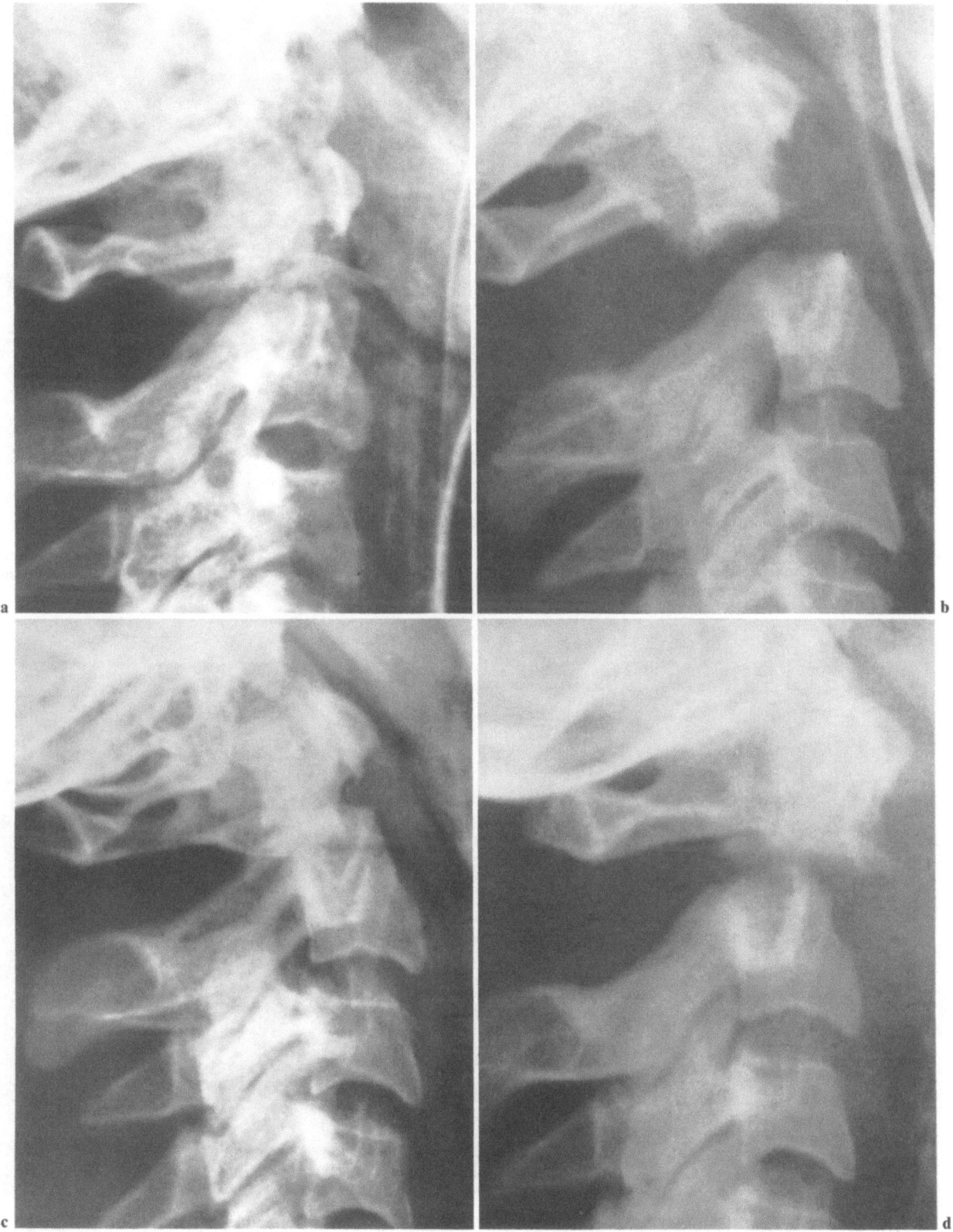

Fig. 21 a–d. English policeman's helmet fracture. The dynamic study shows global instability: **a** in neutral position, rotatory displacement; **b** diastasis in traction; **c** posterior displacement in extension; **d** anterior displacement in flexion

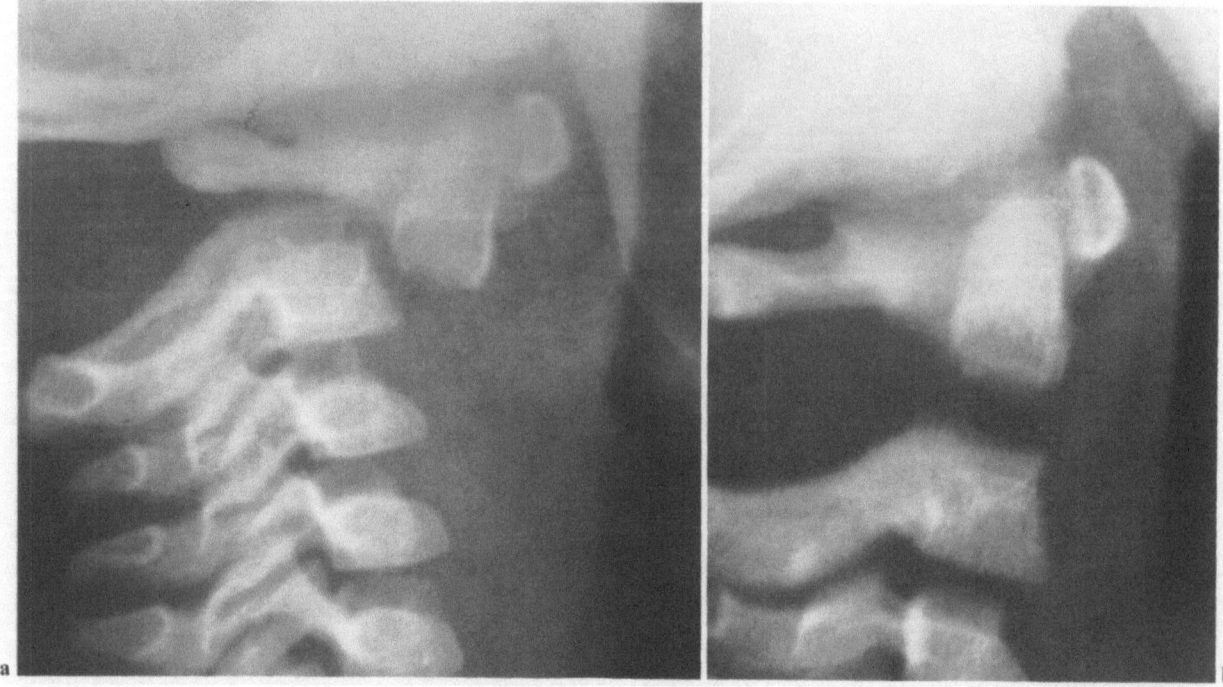

Fig. 22a, b. Acute epiphysiolysis of the odontoid leading to tetraplegia with apparent death. Emergency reduction was followed by almost complete neurologic recuperation. **a** Detachment of the dens. Note the swelling of the prevertebral soft parts; **b** radiograph taken after reduction, extension, and traction

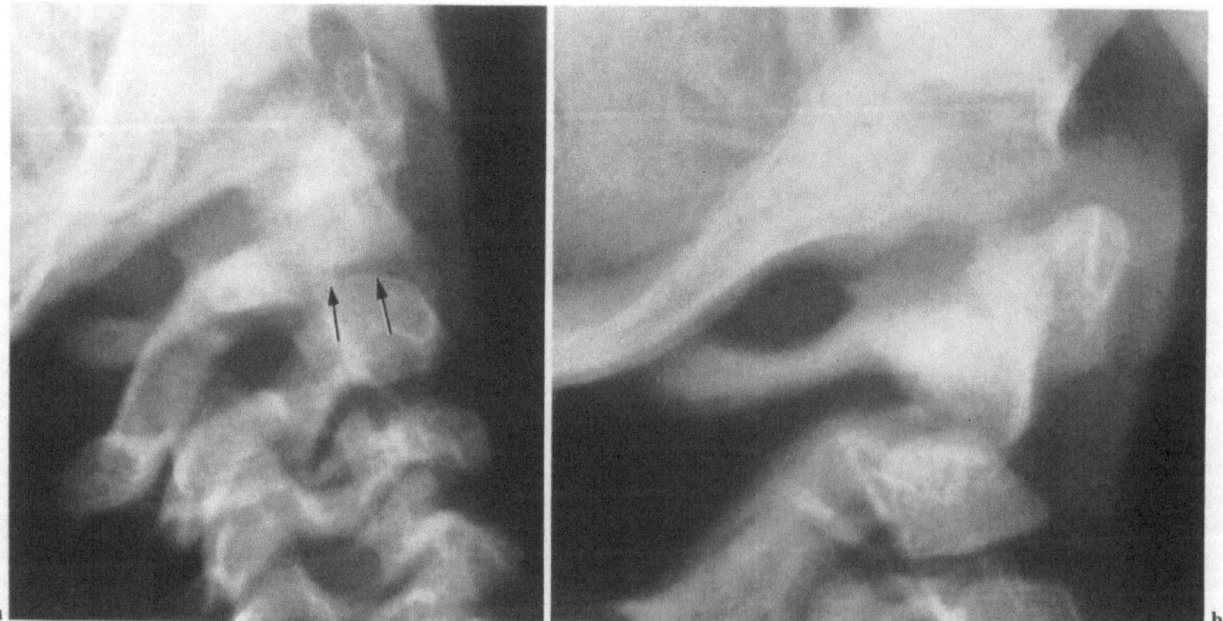

Fig. 23a, b. Progressive epiphysiolysis in a 4½-year-old child that had fallen from the first floor. On the film taken on the day of the accident (**a**) the translucent line between C1 and C2 is identified as the vestigial disk *(arrows)*. No disalignment or thickening of the prevertebral soft parts is seen despite the poor incidence. On the control film taken 30 days later (**b**) because of persistent torticollis the disaligrement. The course was unremarkable after orthopedic treatment

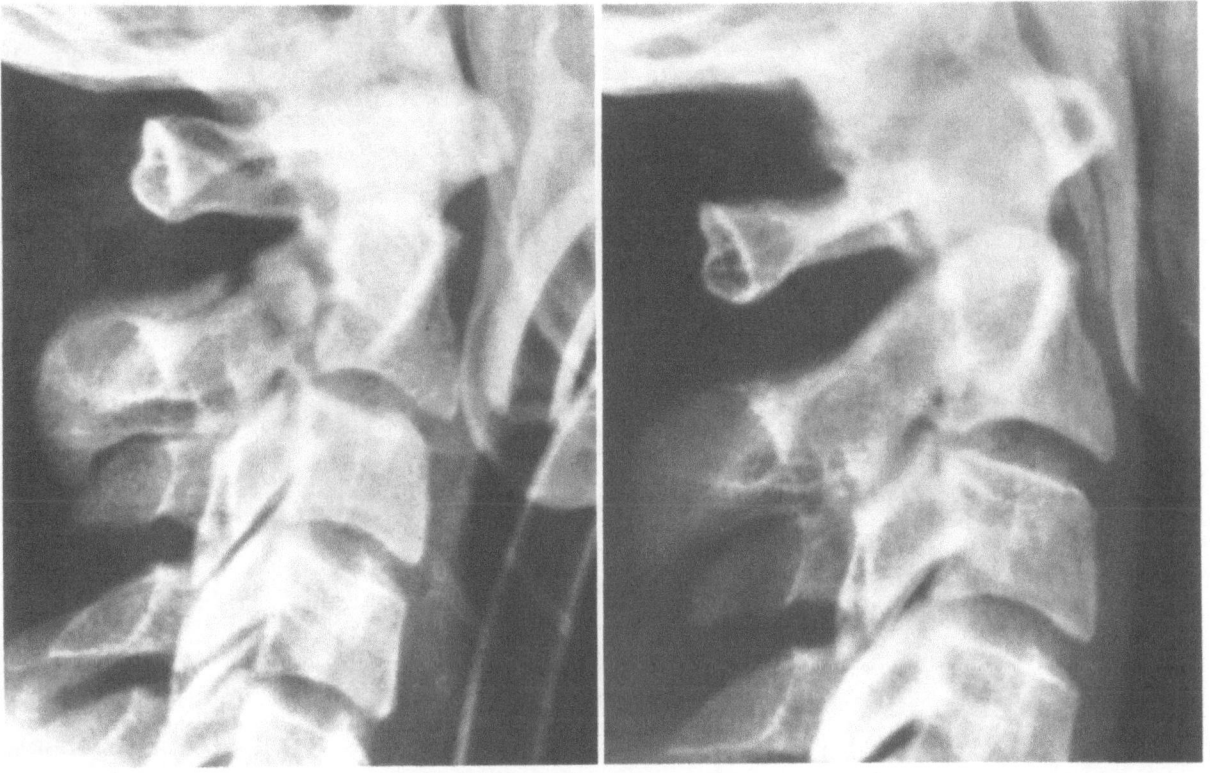

a · b

Fig. 24a, b. Type I fracture of the pedicles of C2 following a traffic accident. No neurologic signs are seen (**a**). The fracture was treated by continuous extension. A check after treatment (**b**) revealed no signs of disk deterioration. This is a stable type I fracture, according to C. LAURIN's classification (EFFENDY et al. 1981)

α) C2–C3 Anterior Disk Instability

This is seen as an abnormal angulation of 11° or more between the C2 and C3 vertebral bodies and/or a listhesis of more than 4 mm between the posterior aspects of C2 and C3, associated with an anterior displacement of the C1–C2 spinous process. With increasing severity of such a sprain these figures become more extreme. The intervertebral disk is considered to be totally destroyed when the listhesis is equal to or more than half the width of the vertebral body. Another important sign of severe sprain is a fracture of the anterosuperior angle of the C2 body. We shall consider its significance for the study of tear-drop fractures of the lower cervical vertebrae.

β) C2–C3 Posterior Interarticular Instability

The following signs are seen on a radiograph:
C1–C2 and C2–C3 interspinous gaping

Forward displacement of the C1–C2 and C2–C3 spinous processes relative to the underlying spinolaminar line
Interarticular dislocation by over 50% and sometimes even C2–C3 posterior luxation

This severe posterior luxation is always accompanied by C2–C3 disk involvement.

LAURIN's studies (EFFENDY et al. 1980) allow schematic consideration of three types of fractures:

Type I Pedicular fracture without discoligamentous instability. This lesion results from compression in hyperextension (Fig. 24).

Type II Pedicular fracture with anterior discoligamentous instability. The C2–C3 posterior interapophyseal articulations are usually intact. The C2/C3 disk instability is global in flexion and in extension. Therefore it is difficult to stabilize the lesion. Actually the treatment consists in arthrodesis by anterior approach. Depending on

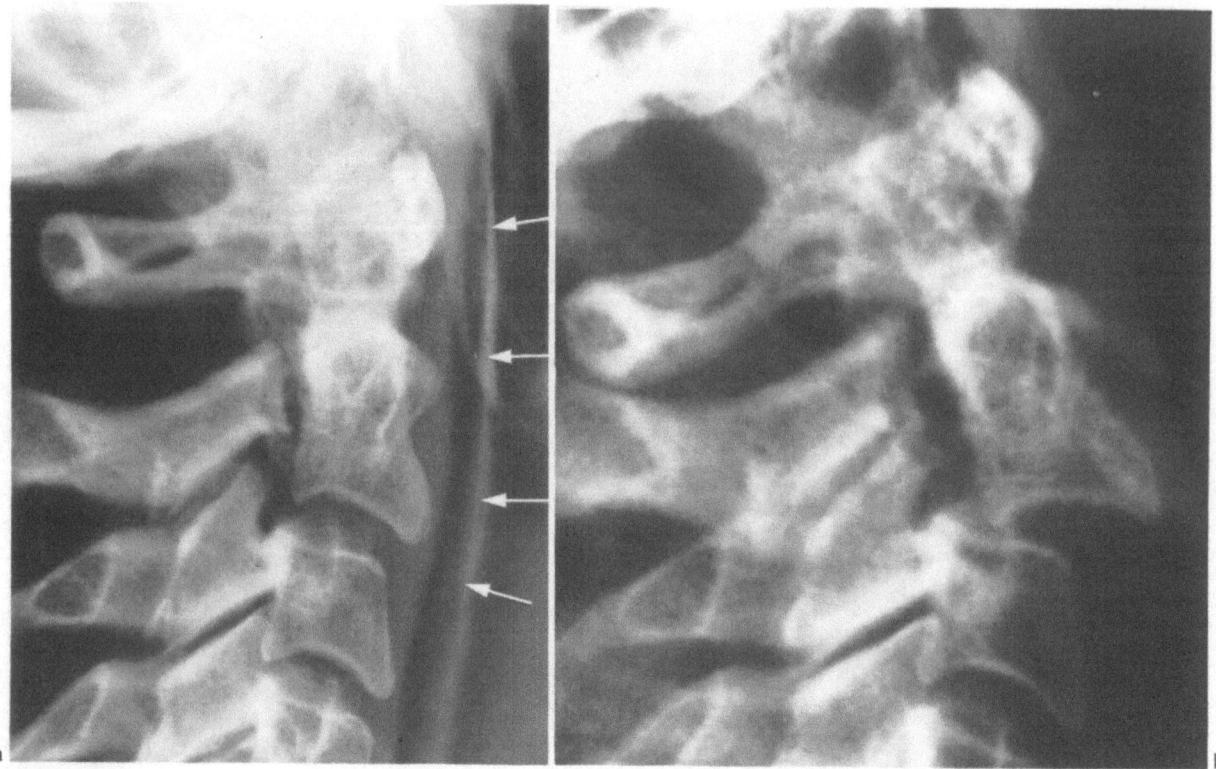

a   b

Fig. 25a, b. Type II fracture of the pedicles of C2. **a** Initial investigation. Following a traffic accident the patient presented with a trauma to the skull and loss of consciousness but no neurologic symptoms. Note the presence of air in the retropharyngeal space due to a pneumomediastinum (MIN-ᴺᴱᴳᴬᴿᴼᴰᴱ's sign; *arrow*). **b** Control film taken after a 1 month's immobilization in a plaster Minerva collar. Secondary displacement of the axis body indicates involvement of the disk and of the longitudinal anterior ligament and increase of the fractural space with possible evolution to pseudarthrosis

whether the major mechanism is hyperflexion or hyperextension, the instability will predominate in the same direction (Fig. 25).

Type III Pedicular fracture with C2–C3 posterior interapophyseal luxation. This lesion with posterior instability is always accompanied by anterior disk instability. It occurs on a spine in hyperflexion, contrariwise to type I. The reduction of the posterior luxation is difficult and often requires surgery. Fixation is in this case even more difficult to obtain (Fig. 26).

The main advantage of the classification based on the factors of instability is help that it is an aid to recognition of the mechanisms causing the lesions (hence their importance in forensic problems) and provides a basis for the treatment.

c) Fractures of the Axis Body

In isolated fractures of the axis body the fracture line is usually oblique and vertical, running poste-

rior to the odontoid base and separating off the third or the anterior part of the axis body. There is usually no displacement. Therefore the diagnosis is difficult on standard projections and tomograms are helpful. Transverse fracture lines are more easily diagnosed, since they are often responsible for a lateral displacement of the upper part of the axis body, which is clearly reveated on a transbuccal view. Fractures within the spongy bone do not cause consolidation problems. We have already seen that this is not the case with corporeal fractures extending either onto the odontoid process or onto the pedicles.

A lesion peculiar to this vertebra occurs when an anteroinferior corner of the axis body is torn off; the mechanism concerned is that of a fracture occurring in hyperextension with involvement of the anterior common vertebral ligament. In contrast to the other cervical vertebrae, where it is responsible for tear-drop fracture with severe

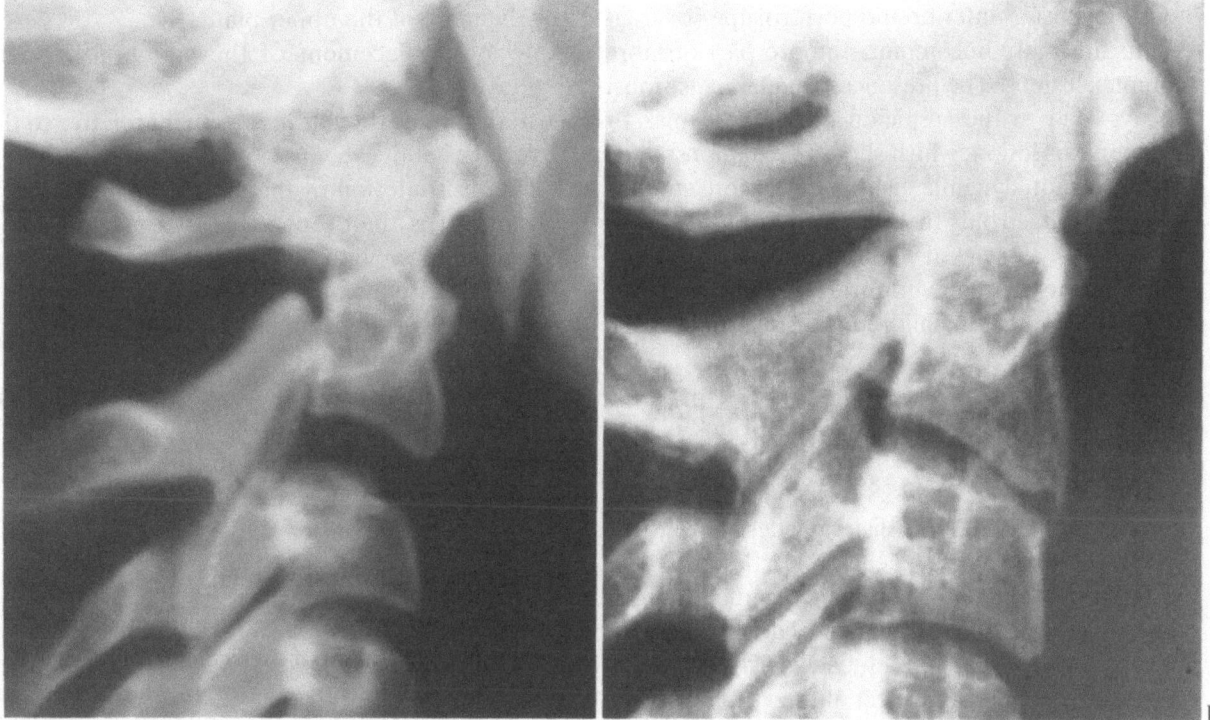

Fig. 26a, b. Type III fracture of the pedicles of C2 (C. Laurin), sustained in a road accident with trauma to the skull, loss of consciousness, no neurologic signs. **a** Bilateral posterior interarticular over the top luxation involving marked widening of the C2–C3 disk space with angulation and moderate antelisthesis. **b** Control film taken 7 months later reveals good stabilization of the anterior and posterior lesions. Note again the posttraumatic degeneration of the C2–C3 disk

anterior and posterior instability, this type of lesion is usually stable at this level and consolidates easily without sequelae.

II. Median and Lower Cervical Segment (C3 to C7)

Investigation of a direct or indirect trauma to the median and lower cervical segment, i.e., to the most mobile segment of the spine, is the main source of the radiologist's timidity, with justification. This timidity is twofold: the radiologist is afraid of aggravating the neurologic damage on the one hand, and on the other of overlooking a vertebral lesion. While diagnosis of fractures of the vertebral bodies is rather easy, we shall see that diagnosis of isolated fractures of the posterior arch or discoligamentous lesions requires especial care.

From the clinical point of view, there is also a marked discrepancy between the functional and the physical signs. Pain and stiffness are usually noted. There is no correlation between their intensity and the patient's neurologic status. Except in comatose patients, clinical examination will reveal some evidence of a neurologic lesion, e.g., cervicobrachial neuralgia, tetraplegia, paraplegia, paresis of the diaphragm, regressive tetraplegia, flaccid paraplegia. We shall analyze in turn the corporeal lesions, the lesions of the posterior arch, and those of the discoligamentous structures.

1. Corporeal Lesions

a) Triangular Vertebral Body Fracture

The fracture line is oblique and short, and detaches a triangular fragment from the vertebral edge. It is usually located on the upper vertebral end-plate. The vertebral body is otherwise intact. There is no wedging for instance. This means that the uninvolved vertebral part has a normal height. An anterosuperior fragment would result from hyperflexion, an anteroinferior fragment from hyperextension. Posteroinferior and posterosuperior fragments are more uncommon and are part of more complex lesions. The presence of such images must always lead to the suspicion of a severe disk or ligamentous lesion, which should be demonstrated by means of dynamic flexion-extension studies. They are indeed only the evidence of bone disinsertion and are associated with rupture of the anterior or posterior common vertebral ligament.

The equivalent in children is disinsertion of the anterior margin.

b) Tear-Drop Fracture

This lesion (Figs. 27 and 28) is also a fracture of a corner, but one feature distinguishes it from the type described above. Its characteristics are:

Tearing-off of a more or less triangular anterior and inferior vertebral fragment. The fracture line runs obliquely down- and backward; it usually begins on the anterior aspect of the vertebral body and extends to the lower vertebral plate.

The vertebral fragment detached in this way remains in alignment with the anterior aspects of the subjacent vertebrae.

The vertebral body is displaced backward so that the AP diameter of the canal is diminished. Because of this displacement the lesion becomes extremely neurotoxic.

The disk is damaged.

Marked capsuloligamentous lesions exist at the level of the posterior arch; they are responsible for a posterior interarticular diastasis with regard to the underlying vertebra.

The mechanism of this lesion is still unknown. Some workers, such as ROY-CAMILLE, consider that it is an involvement of the mobile segment, while others, such as FUENTÈS, see it as a lesion resulting from flexion-compression.

We believe both hypotheses to be correct.

The flexion-compression hypotheses is especially credible in that there are most often other lesions associated, either of the posterior arch or of the vertebra above or below, of the sagittal fracture type. Moreover, the tear-drop fracture is quite frequent in diving accidents. In such a case, if the film is turned upside down the similarities with a lesion resulting from flexion-compression, i.e., tear-drop fracture type I, are striking:

Involvement of the upper plate

Anterior displacement of the vertebral segment above

Posterior interarticular involvement relative to the vertebra above

That it is a lesion of the mobile segment is also possible. It is then secondary to a mechanism in hyperextension with distraction (tear-drop type II). In this case it would be opposed point by point to an intervertebral luxation, which is characterized by:

Avulsion of an anterosuperior corner of the underlying vertebral body

Posterior interarticular involvement or luxation with regard to the vertebra above.

c) Wedge-Compression Fracture

Wedge-compression is seen on a roentgenogram in the diminished height of one aspect of the vertebral body, usually the anterior or the lateral aspect, associated with compression of the bone structure, which thus appears more dense.

Compression can be global, extending from the anterior to the posterior wall, or only partial, i.e., anterior or lateral.

When there is a wedge-compression fracture displacements should be looked for. These can be of different types:

No displacement.

Anterior displacement of the detached fragment due to a transverse fracture line, with an increased AP diameter of the vertebra. Such lesions are usually stable and not neurotoxic.

Posterior displacement of the remaining part of the vertebra with a reduced AP diameter of the canal. This type of fracture, with protrusion of the posterior wall, is most often accompanied by neurologic damage and is unstable.

The degree of compression can be expressed in two ways: either as a percentage or as an angle. This quantification serves as a reference for the orthopedic prognosis. Indeed, even if they have been correctly reduced these lesions leave an intrasomatic vacuum with subsequent secondary compression and kyphosis. The main mechanism in the development of these compressions is an axial compression force bearing upon a flexed spine.

Fig. 27. Tear-drop fracture at the C4–C5 level, with tearing-off of the anteroinferior corner of the C4 body and marked backward displacement of the posterior wall of C4 relative to C5

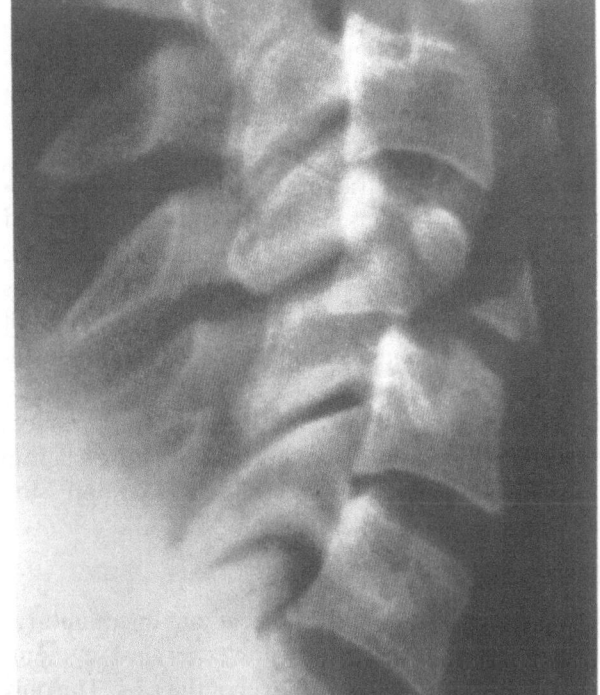

Fig. 28a, b. Multiple injuries in hyperextension. **a** Lateral view shows tearing-off of the inferior part of the anterior arch of the atlas, corresponding to disinsertion of the long muscle of the neck ($\xrightarrow{1}$), tearing-off of the anteroinferior corner of C2 ($\xrightarrow{2}$), and antelisthesis of C6 with slight avulsion of the superior annular epiphysis, undicating a bipedicular fracture-disinsertion ($\xrightarrow{3}$). **b** Control radiograph after orthopedic treatment (5th month) reveals stabilization of the lesions. Note the narrowing of the C5–6 disk space, indicating involvement of this disk in the initial trauma

▽

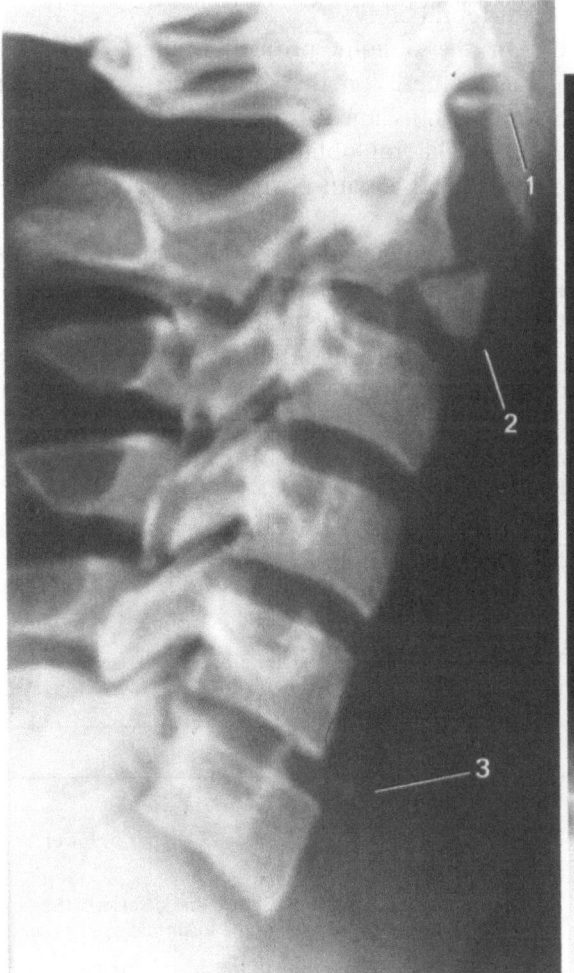

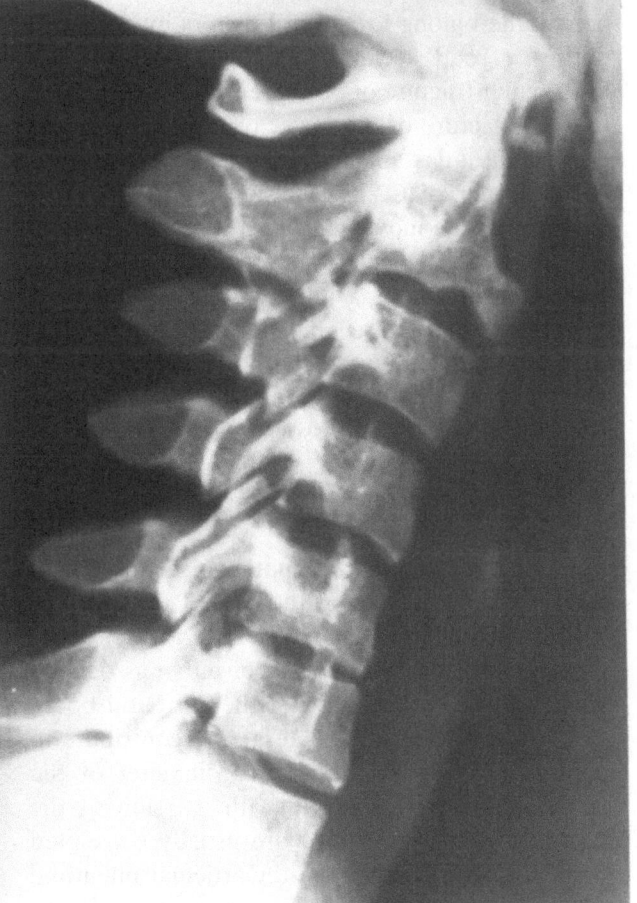

a

b

d) Purely Sagittal Fractures

The lateral radiograph is normal whereas the frontal view shows a vertical intersomatic translucency, which must not be mistaken for the laryngoglottic path.

Purely sagittal fractures are sometimes accompanied by an increase in the transverse diameter of the vertebra, increased interpedicular distance, and swelling of the prevertebral soft tissues. This type of lesion is never seen with reduced height of the vertebral body, so that there is no bone instability.

When the lesions are of minor importance, frontal tomograms may be helpful. Pure sagittal fractures would result from an axial compression force applied to an erect spine.

e) Pedicular Fractures

Isolated fractures of the pedicles are uncommon at the level of the median and lower cervical segment, but more common at the level of the axis. The only case we have seen was in a young woman who had been pulled along for several meters by a vehicle during a road accident (Fig. 28). Besides the bipedicular fracture of C5 there were several other lesions: fracture of the lower part of the anterior arch of the atlas and tearing-off of the anteroinferior corner of C2. The lesions were due to a hyperextension movement. Can we thus conclude that isolated bipedicular fractures are caused by the same mechanism?

This type of fracture is diagnosed on conventional radiograms only when there is a displacement. They then show isolated antelisthesis of a single vertebral body, usually associated with swelling of the prevertebral soft parts, and normal spinolaminar line and alignment of the posterior articular pillars.

When the fragments are not displaced the diagnosis can only be made with axial CT.

Apart from this uncommon case, fractures of the pedicles are more frequently seen either associated with fracture compression of the vertebral body, when they are usually bilateral and contribute to enlarge ment of the transverse diameter of the spinal canal, or associated with a lesion of the posterior arch, when they are usually correlated with fracture-separation of the articular pillar and are unilateral.

2. Lesions of the Posterior Arch

Isolated lesions of the posterior arch have long been overlooked, and they were formerly often only diagnosed after progressing naturaly for some time. They are actually quite common in our daily practice and since we are aware of their existence we hardly try to demonstrate them radiologically. But this awareness should not lead the radiologist to multiply the radiographic and tomographic investigations. Interruptions in the continuity are seldom visible on standard projections and must always be looked for with the aid of tomograms. Usually a strictly lateral projection is enough. Various signs that are visible on the standard projections make tomograms essential; these signs fall into two groups:

1. Lateralized antelisthesis syndrome. This is made up of several signs, i.e.,
a) On the lateral view: moderate antelisthesis of a vertebral body
b) On the oblique projection: increase of the antelisthesis on the same side as the lesion, revealed by uncovertebral gaping
c) Contralateral oblique projection: absence of antelisthesis with normal uncovertebral interspace

Besides the lateral antelisthesis, the frontal projection shows a deviation of the spinous process toward the side of the lesion.

The syndrome of lateralized antelisthesis associated with deviation of the spinous process is, to us, a sign revealing the presence of a lesion of the posterior articular pillar or of the means of union between the pillars.

We shall see later the lesional significance of this for the lesion (Table 2).

Table 2. Classification of lateralized antelisthesis into four types

Type	Anatomical lesions
Type I	Unilateral luxation
Type II	Fracture of articular process (upper or lower)
Type III	Fracture of the isthmus In this variety the fracture line disinserts the upper articular process from the lower articular process
Type IV	Fracture-separation of the articular pillar

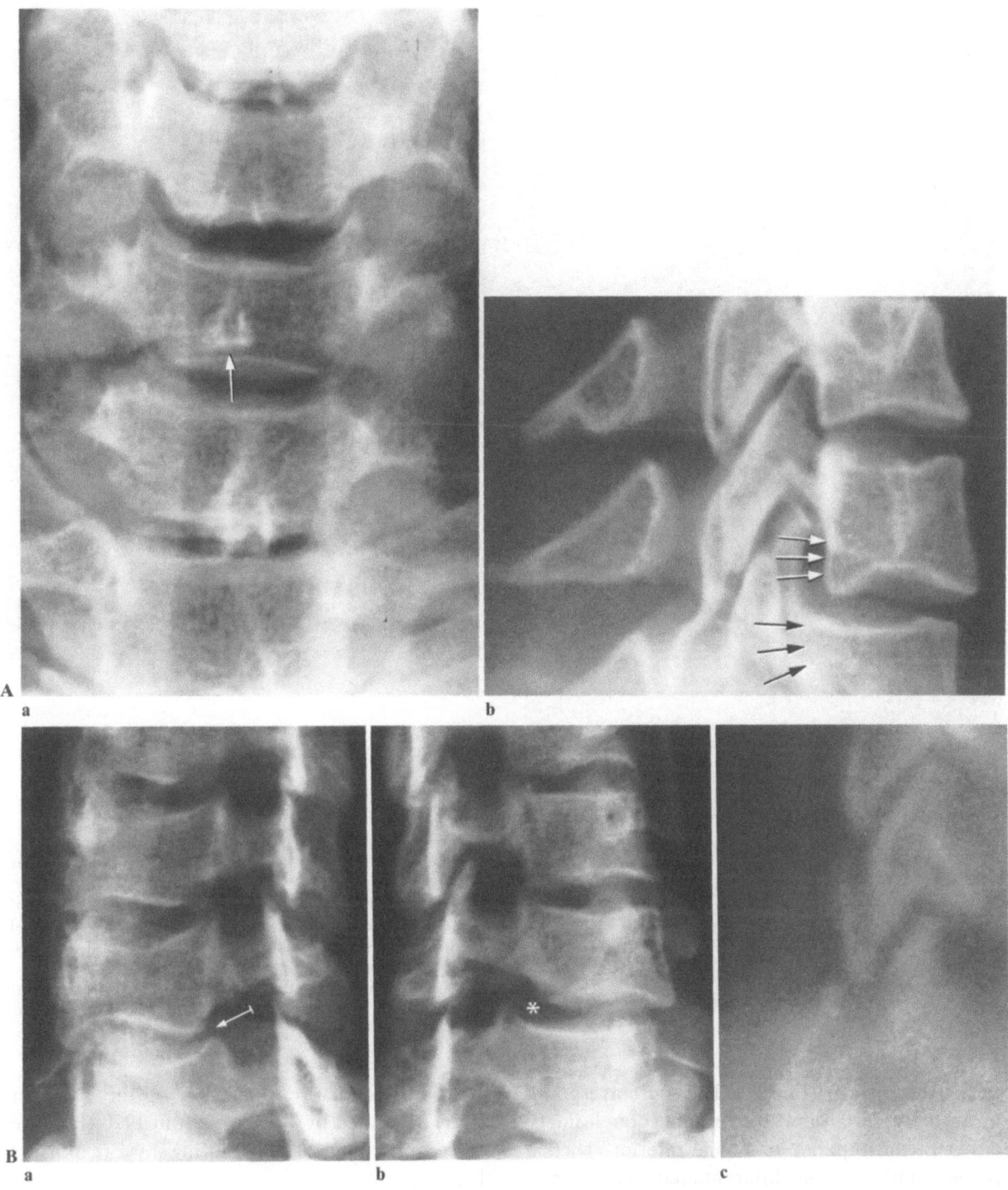

Fig. 29 A, B. Lateralized antelisthesis syndrome: fracture of the right pars interarticularis of C6.
Aa Frontal view: deviation of the spinous process on the injured side (→). **b** Lateral view: C6–C7 antelisthesis (⇉).
Ba Right posterior oblique projection with normal left uncover-

tebral joint (↦). **b** Left posterior oblique projection with right uncovertebral gaping (∗). **c** Tomogram reveals fracture of the pars interarticularis with normal posterior interarticular connections. The antelisthesis is due to a fracture displacement and not to the luxation as in the case of Fig. 39

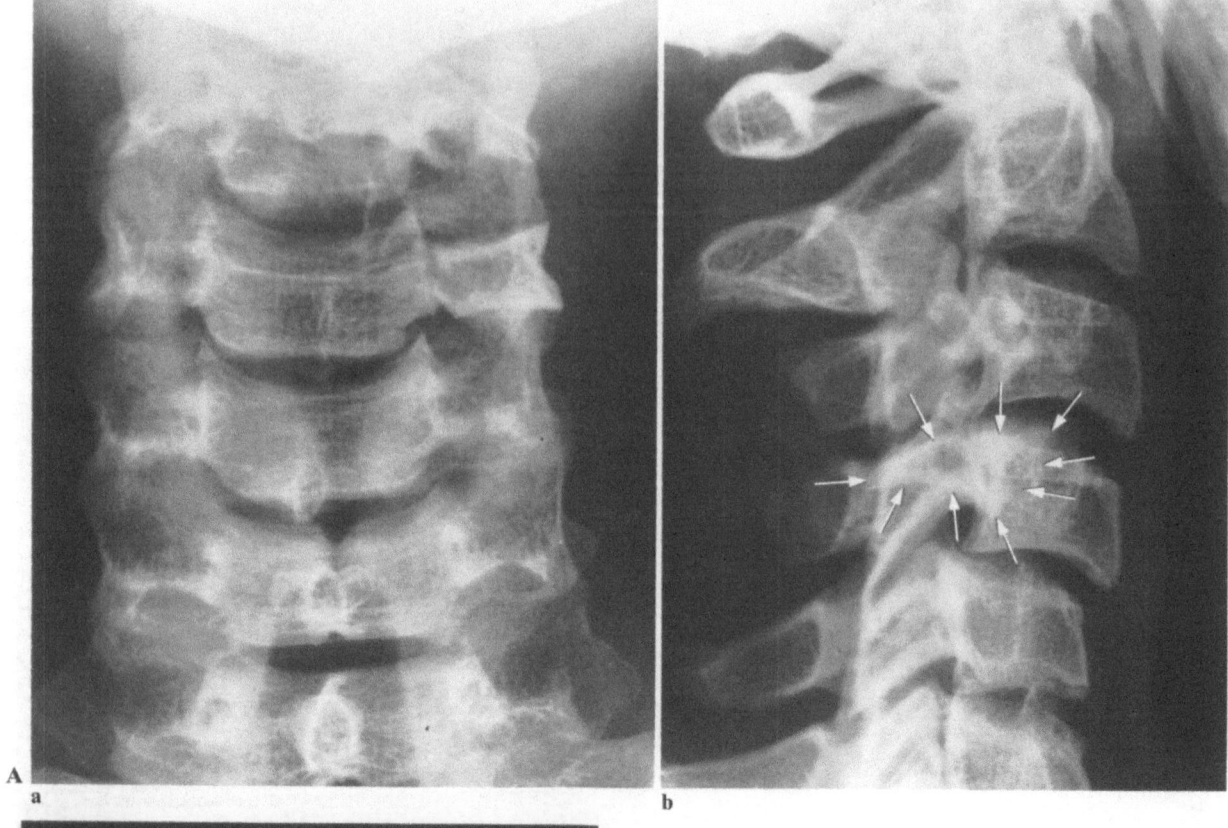

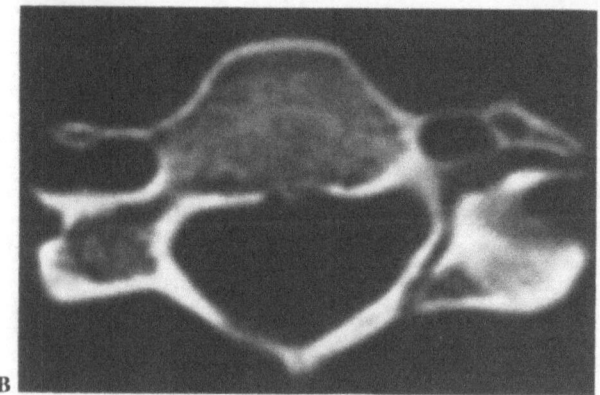

Fig. 30 A, B. Sagittal avulsion-fracture of the left articular pillar of C4.
A Radiologic images: **a** frontal view: the left articular pillar of C4 is rectangular with the long axis transverse (in normal articular processes the long axis is vertical); **b** lateral view: the *arrows* delineate the injured and tilted articular process.
B CT investigation shows that the fracture of the articular pillar is sagittal. The bony structure of the spinal canal is undamaged

2. "Bow tie" sign (Fig. 31). This sign corresponds on a strictly lateral view to an isolated double image either of the superior or of the inferior articular process and must be differentiated from a combined double image of the upper and lower articular process. The latter is a sign of a discrete rotation or inclination (Fig. 32).

a) Fracture-Separation of the Articular Pillar

Depending on the causative mechanism we recognize two different types of fractures:

Type I: Fracture-separation of the articular pillar, described by JUDET et al. in 1970 (fracture by compression, usually during hyperextension (Fig. 33).

This lesion is usually unilateral and comprises two fracture lines: a posterior one at the level of the lamina and an anterior one on the pedicle. The articular pillar is thus released from its bony attachments and undergoes an anterior tilting motion relative to the transverse axis. This tilting motion varies in the degree of violence and can even

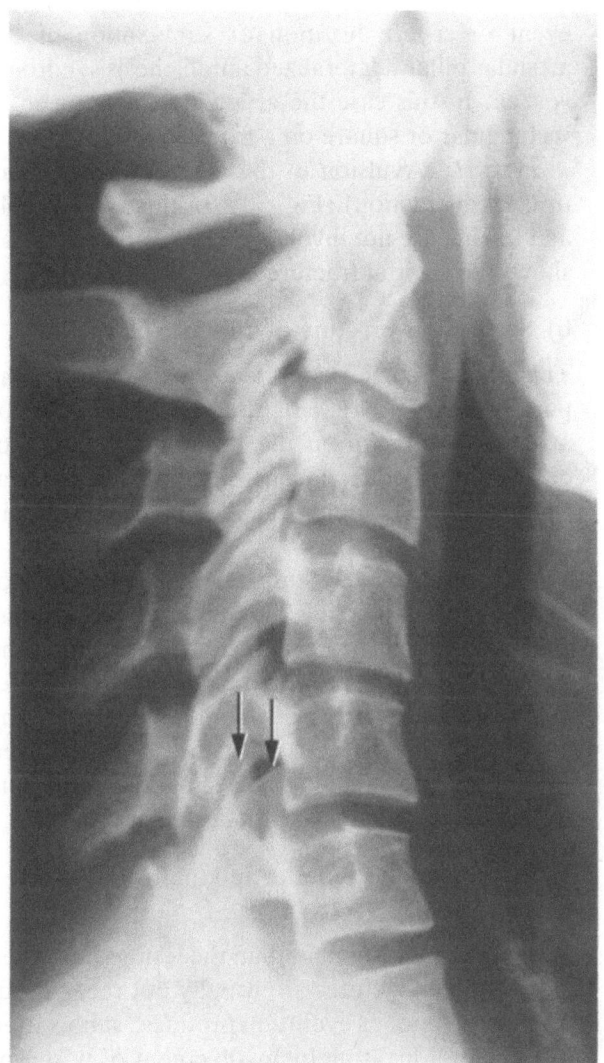

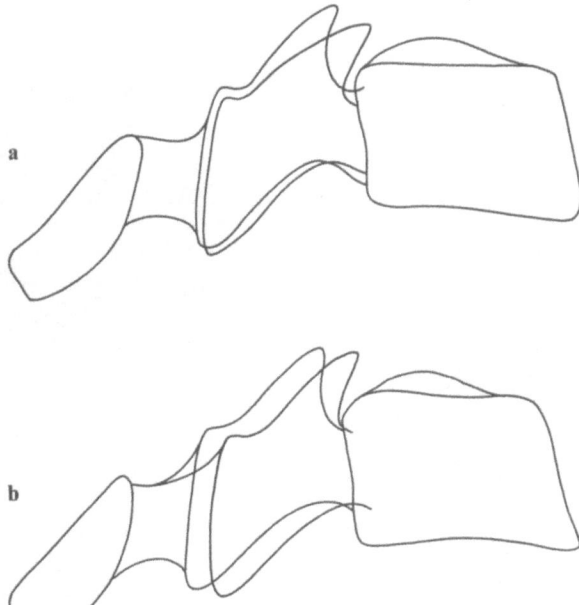

Fig. 32a, b. Bow-tie sign. Schematic representation differentiating between a true **(a)** and a false **(b)** sign

◁
Fig. 31. Bow tie sign. A double image of the superior articular pillars (→) of C6 is seen, corresponding to an isolated fracture of the right superior articulaire pillar. (Clinical investigation revealed cervicobrachial neuralgia)

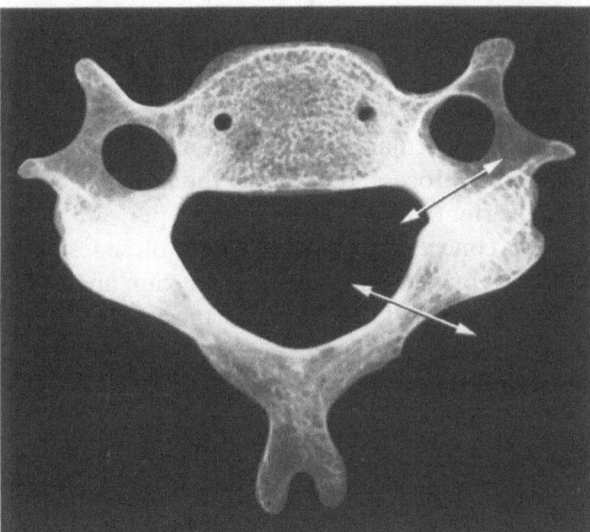

Fig. 33. Fracture-separation of the articular pillar. The *arrows* show the anterior and posterior fractures

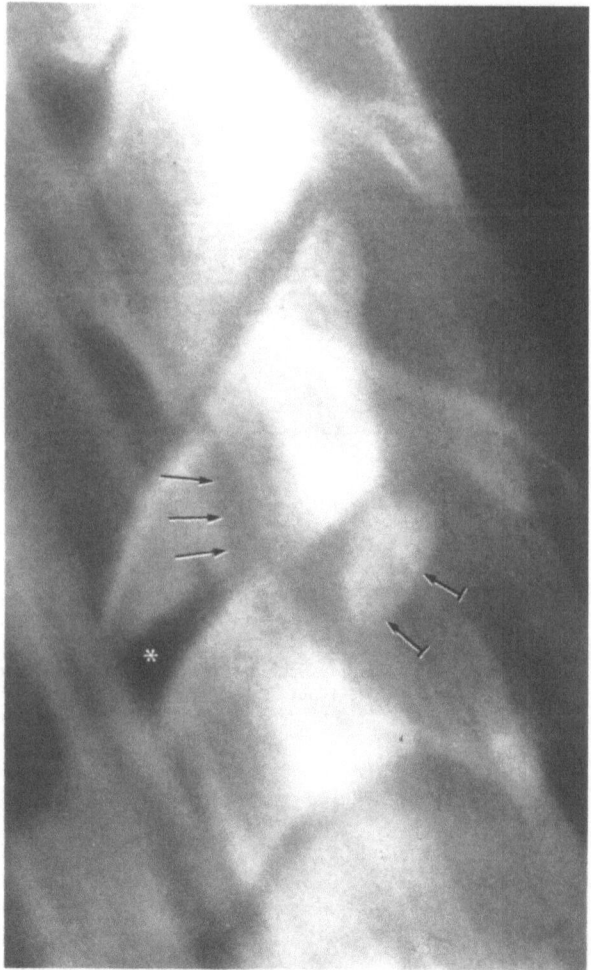

Fig. 34. Lateral tomogram centered on C4–5 and revealing decapitation of the superior articular process of C5 (↦), and transarticular fracture of C4 with disinsertion of a posteroinferior fragment from the articular pillar of C4 (→). Note the posterior interarticular divergence (∗)

produce luxation with rupture of the capsuloligamentous insertions. The pedicular and laminar fracture lines are usually easily visible on oblique projections.

The amplitude of the displacement of the articular pillar determines the nature of the X-ray image.

With simple tilting the frontal view shows an abnormal visibility of the posterior articular interspace, due to a horizontal orientation of the articular pillar. The lateral view reveals a double image of the articular pillars, and the fractured part of the lamina can be seen in the interspinous space. Besides the pedicular and laminar fracture lines, the main feature revealed by an oblique view is the reduced size of the intervertebral foramen. In the

event of severe luxation or subluxation of the articular pillar a lateralized antelisthesis syndrome is seen. In this case the articular pillar is seen as rectangular or square on a frontal view.

Type II: Avulsion of the articular pillar (fracture by distraction) (Fig. 30). In this type pedicle and lamina are not involved. The CT investigation shows the sagittal fracture line.

b) Separation-Fracture of the Articular Pillar

This fracture corresponds in fact to a fracture of the pars interarticularis. It detaches the superior articular process from the inferior articular process, although their means of union and correlations with the homologs above and below remain intact.

When there is no displacement, the diagnosis is almost impossible on standard projections. A 15–20° oblique projection (Fig. 2) will reveal the fracture line on the pars interarticularis in this case.

When there is a displacement there is a striking lateralized antelisthesis on the side involved (Fig. 29). Lateral tomograms show this syndrome to be due to a fracture of the articular pillar.

c) Fracture of the Superior and Inferior Articular Processes

Although more frequent than the lesions described above, these fractures are usually not recognized. Their spontaneous evolution produces subluxation or unilateral luxation by involvement of posterior interarticular means of union. This is particularly so with fractures of the superior articular processes. From the surgical point of view, it is also important to distinguish these two types of fractures. While a direct surgical approach to the inferior articular process is possible, the superior articular process, covered by the articular pillar of the vertebra above, lies much deeper.

As concerns the biomechanics, these lesions are caused by mechanism in lateroflexion and/or rotation, associated with flexion in the case of the upper articular process, and with extension in that of the lower articular process (Fig. 34).

a) Fracture of the Superior Articular Process

The usually oblique fracture line (Fig. 35) is located at a variably high level and realizes a cut-off. The diagnosis of such isolated fractures is difficult and always requires lateral and oblique tomograms to display the fracture lines.

The following signs draw attention to such lesions:

Reduced size of an intervertebral foramen at a single level on the oblique projection.

Bow-tie sign: duplication of the left and right superior articular facets on a lateral view, whereas the posterior aspects of the articular pillars and the inferior articular processes remain superimposed. This image is called the bow-tie sign or batwing appearance. It must be distinguished from the image caused by a slight rotation in which the left and right articular pillars are globally shifted.

Lateralized antelisthesis. The presence of this sign confirms a fracture-displacement or an associated subluxation or luxation.

For all these cases lateral tomographic projections are indispensable. In our daily practice, the existence of cervicobrachial neuralgia is the clinical symptom that most frequently alerts the radiologist.

β) Fracture of the Inferior Articular Process

The radiologic approach is the same as in the previous case. It is very important to recognize this type of fracture, which is usually clinically and radiologically silent.

d) Fracture of the Lamina

Fractures of the lamina is exceptional. We have encountered only one case with bilateral involvement, associated with a luxation. Thanks to the aperture of the posterior arch caused by the luxation, the spinal cord remained unaffected and the patient had no neurologic deficit.

e) Fracture of the Spinous Processes

This fracture involves predominantly the spinous process of C7: it is called the clay-shoveler's fracture and is caused either by a direct impact or by a flexion-extension movement. Its diagnosis is usually easy either on frontal or on lateral radiographs.

3. Sprains and Luxations

Sprains or luxations are caused by lesions of the discoligamentous means of union, i.e., the mobile vertebral segment. They usually result from a purely flexion and/or extension mechanism in the case of bilateral lesions, associated with lateral flexion and rotation in case of unilateral lesion. Such changes seldom occur in isolation usually being associated with bone lesions. They have two main characteristics: instability and the likelihood of neurologic damage. The likelihood of causing neurologic damage is immediate in case of luxation, and progressive in case of an unrecognized, neglected or badly treated benign or severe sprain. The instability is significant, increasing in intensity from benign to severe sprain and to luxation. Instability is immediate and persists while ever the means of union has not healed; healing is difficult to obtain in the absence of strict immobilization, and orthopedic treatment with a plaster collar usually proves in adequate.

a) Luxations

α) Bilateral Luxation

Bilateral luxation is defined by complete rupture of all means of union (interspinous ligament, ligamentum flavum, interarticular ligaments, posterior longitudinal ligament, intervertebral disk and possibly, anterior longitudinal ligament), with a total loss of articular connections. When the posterior longitudinal ligament is not involved there is no luxation.

Clinically, there is a trauma to the spine with neurologic disturbances (complete or incomplete tetraplegia, motor disturbances, etc.).

Neurologic investigations aimed at the detection of a sublesional syndrome must be very thorough, since the findings are of paramount importance for the prognosis. As a matter of fact, complete tetraplegia with abolished motoricity and sublesional sensibility is the most likely to remain complete, and any degree of functional recovery can only be expected when the metameres are not completely involved, at the upper limit of sensorimotor disturbances. Cowersely, incomplete tetraplegia with, for instance, persistence of sphincter reflexes has the best chance of neurologic improvement. Recovery is earlier and sensitivity greater when surgical reduction has been performed early. Therefore, the clinical and radiologic investigations should be brief and accurate to avoid any delay in instituting the initial treatment. Since the radiologic diagnosis is usually easy the initial study requires only two standard projections (one lateral

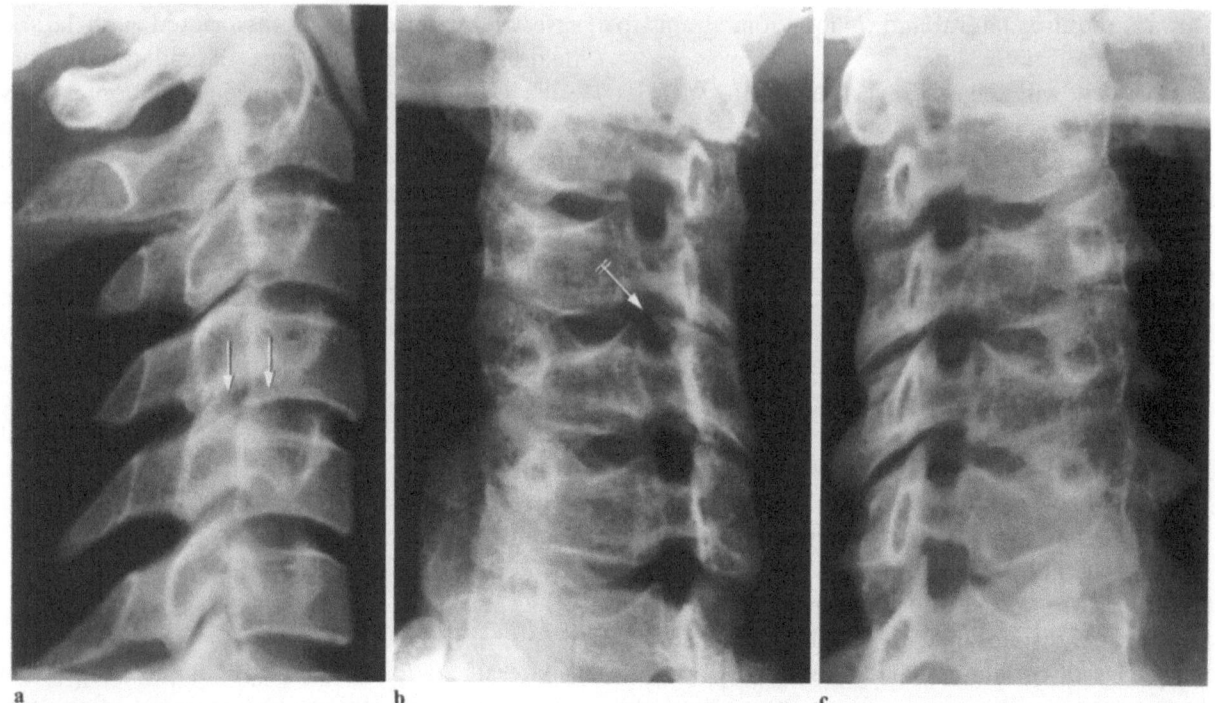

Fig. 35 a–c

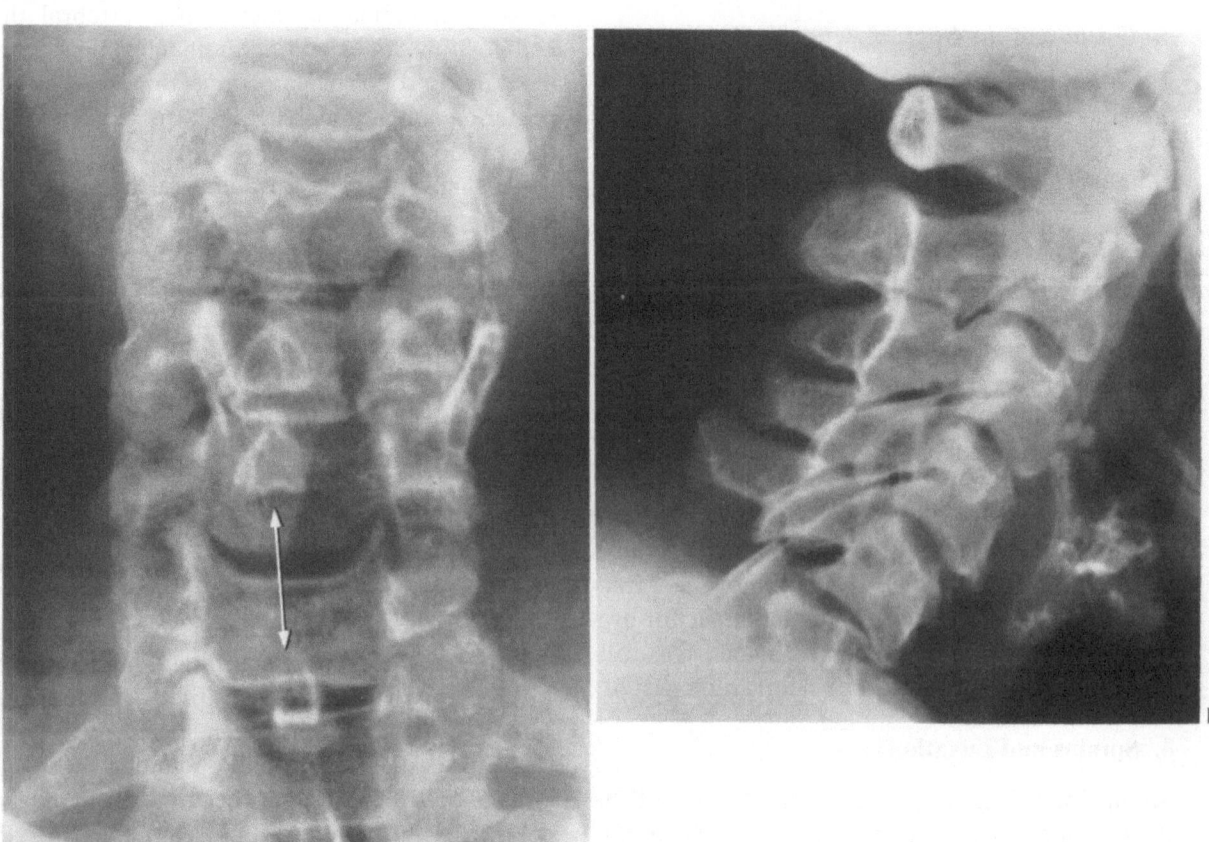

Fig. 36 a, b

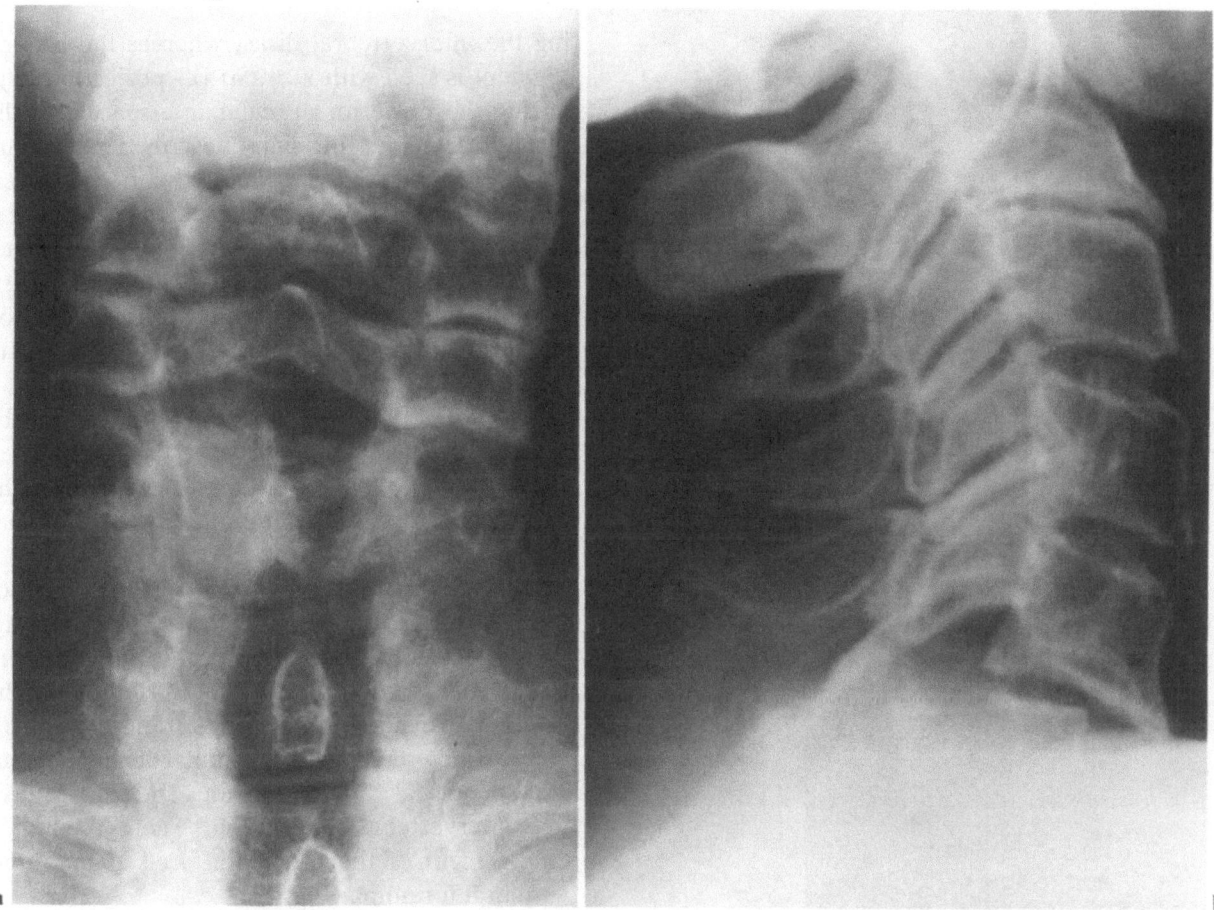

Fig. 37a, b. C5–C6 luxation after a fall due to paresia in the lower limbs. Radiographic investigation was performed 5 days after the accident. Note on the frontal view **(a)** the increased C5–C6 interspinous distance, and especially the difference in the incidence on each side of the luxation. Quadriplegia and postoperative death followed. **b** Lateral view

◁ **Fig. 35a–c.** Fracture of the left superior articular process of C5. **a** Lateral view taken on admission to hospital: the lesion was overlooked in spite of the bow-tie image in C5 (→). **b** On the control film taken 7 days later because of a persistent cervico-brachial neuralgia left and right oblique projections show markedly reduced left C4–C5 intervertebral foramen, due to tilting of the fractured superior articular process (⊦⊦→). **c** The oter side is shown for comparison

◁ **Fig. 36a, b.** C5–C6 luxation on the top in an arthritic spine. The mechanism of injury is hyperflexion; the patient fell backward after feeling faint. Left cervico-brachial neuralgia was recorded. Besides the interspinous gaping (↔), which is easily visible on the frontal view **(a)**, note on the lateral view **(b)** the hypervisibility of the C5–C6 intervertebral foramen. Normally only the C7–T1 intervertebral foramen is visible on a lateral view

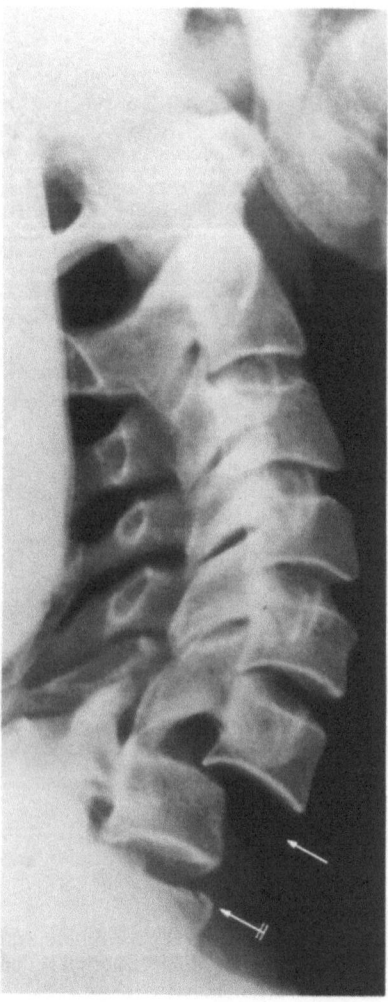

Fig. 38. C6–C7 luxation over the top without lesion of the posterior arch. Tetraplegia was present. Note the torn-off anterosuperior corner of C7 (→) and the parcellar fracture of that of T1 (⊢→)

and one frontal) even if further radiologic investigations are carried out after reduction. The radiologic signs of a luxation are easily recognized. On a *frontal projection*, the interspinous distance is widened on the midline, at the level of the luxated vertebra, and at the suprajacent level there is a narrowing of this distance or even contact between the spinous processes (Fig. 36). On the pedicular lines the gaping is accompanied by an increased interpedicular distance between two adjacent vertebrae.

Other, no less important, signs can be recognized. There is a brisk disparity in the type of incidence. Thus, the lower cervical spine is seen with the 20° ascendant standard incidence visualiz-

ing the intervertebral disks, whereas the luxated segment is seen with DORLAND's projection visualizing the posterior articular interspaces. In the luxated segment the signs described above are again encountered, with marked corporeal overlapping (Fig. 37). When this incidence disparity is brisk and appears between two adjacent vertebrae, it is pathognomonic for a top luxation. In contrast, when the transition is progressive its interpretation should be more critical. It can then also be due to inversion in the sagittal curvature, usually associated with pseudospondylolisthesis caused by arthrosis.

The *lateral projection* allows correction of the diagnosis and permits differentiation of two types of luxation.

In *type I,* or luxation on the top, the posterior articular interspace is completely revealed and the inferior articular process of the luxated vertebra remains suspended on the superior aspect of the superior articular process of the underlying vertebra, which remains in position. The interspinous and uncodiskal gaping is obvious and causes maximal intervertebral angulation. There is also an enlargement of the projection area of the intervertebral foramina (Fig. 37).

In *type II,* or luxation over the top, the luxated inferior articular process is located in front of the anterior aspect of the superior articular process of the underlying vertebra. In this case the interspinous and uncodiskal widening is less obvious, and the intervertebral foramina may bve narrowed. The intervertebral angulation is less marked and instead significant antelisthesis is seen (Fig. 38).

It is very important for the surgeon to be able to recognize these two varieties of luxation. Indeed, while luxation on the top does not cause problems with reduction, luxation over the top is sometimes more difficult to treat and may even require surgery.

Luxations seldom occur in isolation, generally being associated with bony lesions that must also be diagnosed. These lesions are of two kinds, and vary in significance depending on whether they are located on the anterior column or on the posterior neural arch.

Anterior Lesions. Avulsion of the anterosuperior corner of the underlying vertebra is associated with

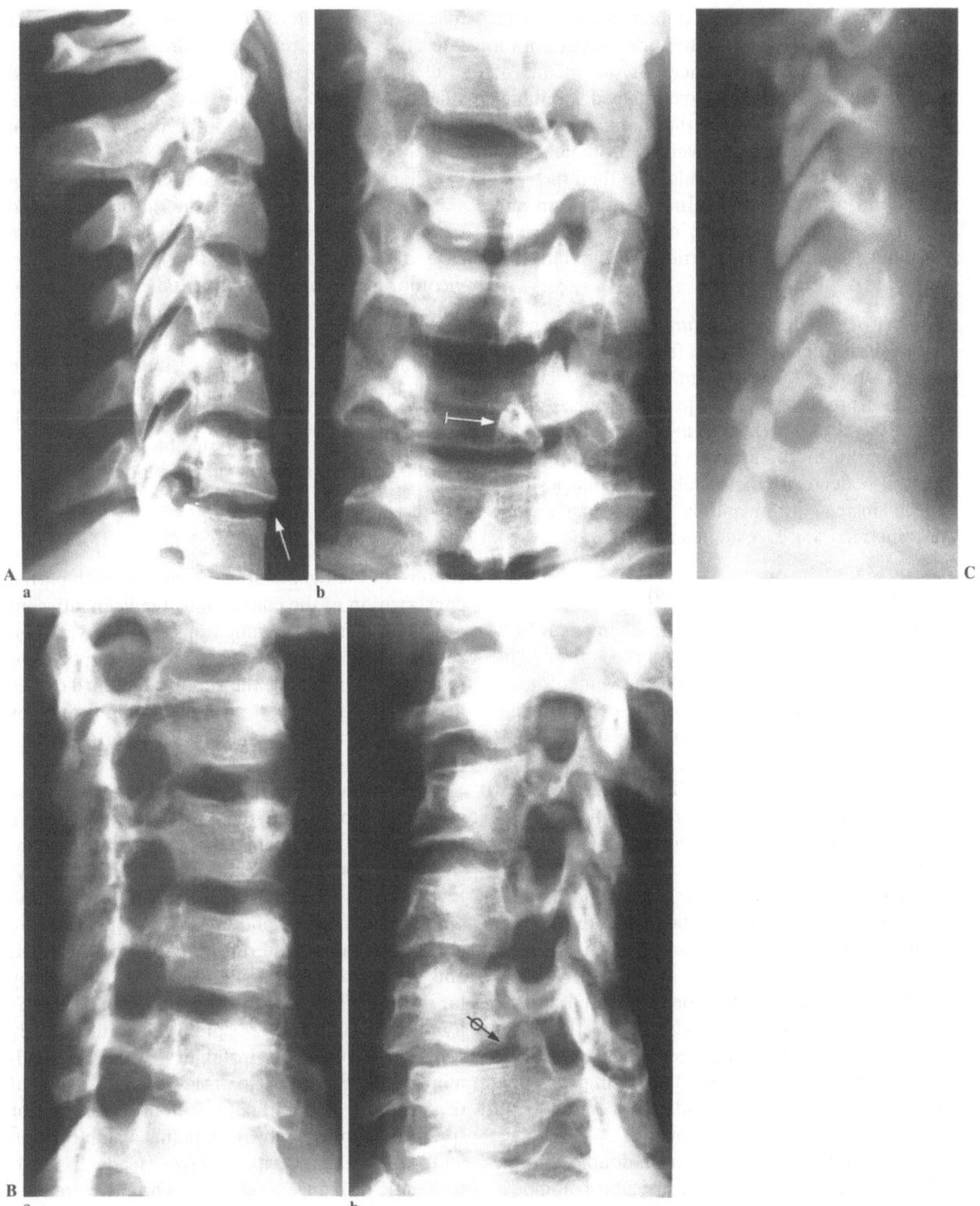

Fig. 39 A–C. Unilateral luxation with lateralized antelisthesis syndrome:

A a lateral view: C5–C6 antelisthesis (→); **b** frontal view: deviation of the spinous process on the side of the lesion (↦).
B a Left posterior oblique projection showing that the various intervertebral connections are normal; **b** right posterior oblique projection revealing left uncovertebral gaping (↔).
C Tomogram reveals unilateral luxation with cut-off of the articular process

marked swelling of the prevertebral soft parts. This sign should always attract attention and prompt a search for severe involvement of the means of union. The luxation may have reduced spontaneously and not be seen on the initial roentgenograms. In a patient with severe neurologic symptoms such as tetraplegia, avulsion is then the only indication of the luxation. In older children and young adults, in whom the annular epiphysis is becoming ossified, disinsertion of the latter is observed.

Lesions of the Posterior Neural Arch. Lesions of the posterior neural arch are frequently associated with fractures of the articular processes, laminae, or spinous processes. Their presence causes opening of the neural arch, thus avoiding cord damage by a shearing mechanism in some cases. Moreover, they also decrease the instability of the lesions, which instead from purely being ligamentous become mixed, i.e., osteoligamentous.

β) Unilateral Luxations (Fig. 39)

Unilateral luxations are more frequent than bilateral ones, but they are often not recognized. The mechanism is a hyperflexion movement with lateroflexion and rotation, such as occurs during traffic accidents due to anterolateral shock. Clinically they are well tolerated, but they can cause damage to the nerve roots. Therefore a cervical trauma with a radicular syndrome of the cervicobrachial neuralgia type or radicular palsy should suggest a unilateral luxation.

There are several radiologic signs; some of them, for instance lateralized antelisthesis, are specific, while others are less so but serve nevertheless to attract attention.

On the frontal projection, on the luxated side the uncovertebral distance is widened and there is a unilateral increase in the interpedicular distance between the luxated and the underlying vertebra. This latter sign suggests consideration of on the top luxation in the differential diagnosis.

On the lateral projection a brisk double contour of the left and right posterior articular columns is seen, the luxated side being projected anteriorly onto the vertebral body. This bayonet sign of the articular columns is specific and pathognomonic. Unfortunately it is difficult to interpret and can be mistaken for a technical error, i.e., incorrect lateral view or vertebral rotation.

On the oblique projection, while the unaffected side has a normal radioanatomy, on the side of the luxation widening of the intervertebral foramen and laminar line disalignment are seen.

When two or three of the above signs are observed together tomograms should be performed to provide evidence of unilateral luxation. In the case of lesions located at the level of the cervicothoracic joint radiographs taken during manual or autotraction, or even to tomograms, may be required for detection.

Treatment of unilateral luxations is easy when the diagnosis has been made early, but it becomes hazardous when the lesion is intractable, complicated by fibrosis, and irreducible. In this event more aggressive surgery will be required.

b) Sprains

A sprain is defined as an elongation or a partial rupture of the ligamentous structures, with partial conservation of the connections between adjacent articular surfaces. Ligamentous damage varies in severity but never involves the strong posterior longitudinal ligament, the rupture of which causes luxation. In the case of a simple sprain it remains intact and ensures immediate intervertebral stability.

The mechanism of the accident must always be assessed. Most often the lesion is caused by a hyperflexion movement followed by hyperextension, thus resulting in the classic whiplash injury. Hyperflexion is responsible for the damage to the posterior ligaments and hyperextension for the anterior sprains (anterior longitudinal ligament and intervertebral disk). Posterior sprains are by far the most frequent, and depending on the severity of the lesions (severe sprain), lead to a slowly progressive secondary instability, which may culminate in luxation due to progressive stretching of the posterior longitudinal ligament. The anterior sprain, in contrast, always remains a stable lesion and, depending on its severity, leads to posttraumatic disk degeneration which may culminate in arthrosis and functional block.

These notions should be well known. The main occasion of this type of lesion is the traffic accident with frontal or posterior impact.

Clinically, benign and severe sprains cause cervicalgiae and an electively painful interspinous spot which should always be searched for. This area of exquisite pain is usually located at the bruised intervertebral level. The clinical signs are not always so characteristic, however. Depending on the location of the sprain, the clinical signs may be misleading. This is particularly so in the case of lesions involving the upper cervical spine or the cervicothoracic joint. At these sites the irritation of the posterior branch of the spinal nerves produces a MAIGNE's syndrom; in the case of upper cervical segment lesions, occipital cephalagiae radiating anteriorly or even retro-orbital pain of the type knwon as ARNOLD's neuralgia; and in that of lesions in the cervicothoracic joint, thoracic pains extending to the spinal margin of the scapula.

Finally, there may also be other signs, such as vertigo, hypoacusia, ocular disturbances, and psychosomatic manifestations without objective neurologic symptoms.

In fact only the functional radiologic investigation makes the diagnosis possible. Once a bone lesion has been excluded by means of the standard investigation, flexion-extension functional studies are justified as soon as the first day. These studies are performed under the radiologist's surveillance, the amplitude of the active movements being limited by the pain.

α) Severe Posterior Sprain (Fig. 42 b)

Four fundamental signs permit recognition of a severe posterior sprain. These are:

Abnormally wide interspinous gaping.

Intervertebral angle of over 11°. This angle is measured between the anterior aspects but above all between the posterior aspects of the vertebral bodies, and is found again at the level of the posterior articular interlines, which show a divergence with a posterior angle of the same size.

More than half of the articular surfaces is exposed.

Moderate antelisthesis of more than 2 mm in the lower cervical spine, and more than 4 mm for the cervical spine above C4.

These signs are more reliable in that they can be seen on films taken in the neutral position, recognized by the horizontal CHAMBERLAIN's line and are increased by the flexion and partly reduced by

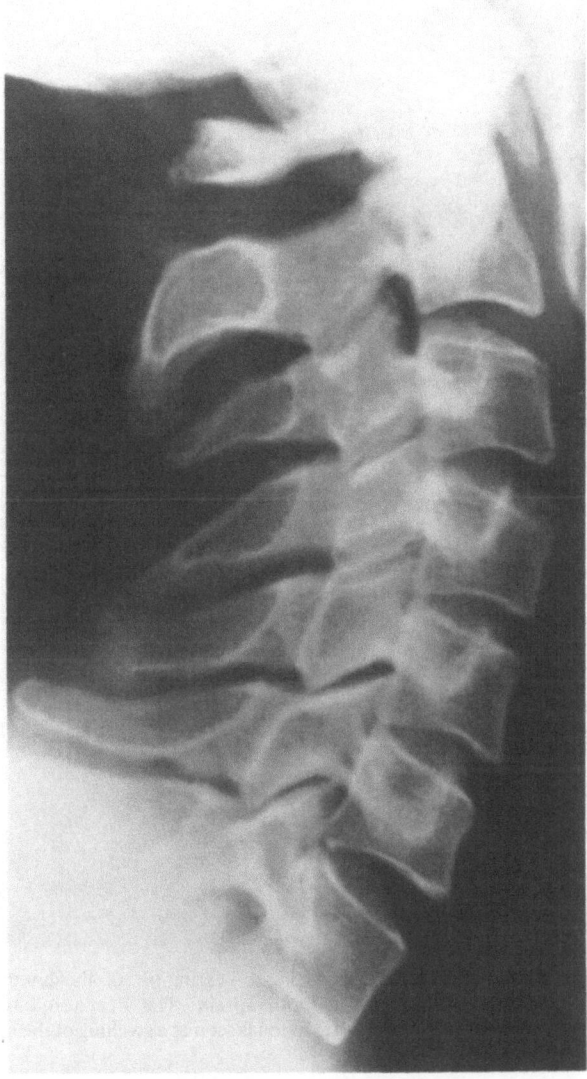

Fig. 40. Anterior whip-lash injury with involvement of the anterior vertebral ligament causing anterior widening of the C6–C7 interspace

extension even on the initial radiograms. But because of the initial muscular contractures, they can also be masked or absent. It is then recommended that the dynamic studies are repeated on the third or fourth day, after palliation of the factors causing the pain.

β) Benign Posterior Sprain

The results of the radiologic investigation remains quasi-normal. The dynamic studies show either overall or segmental rigidity of the cervical spine, or a moderate angular kyphosis, but they never

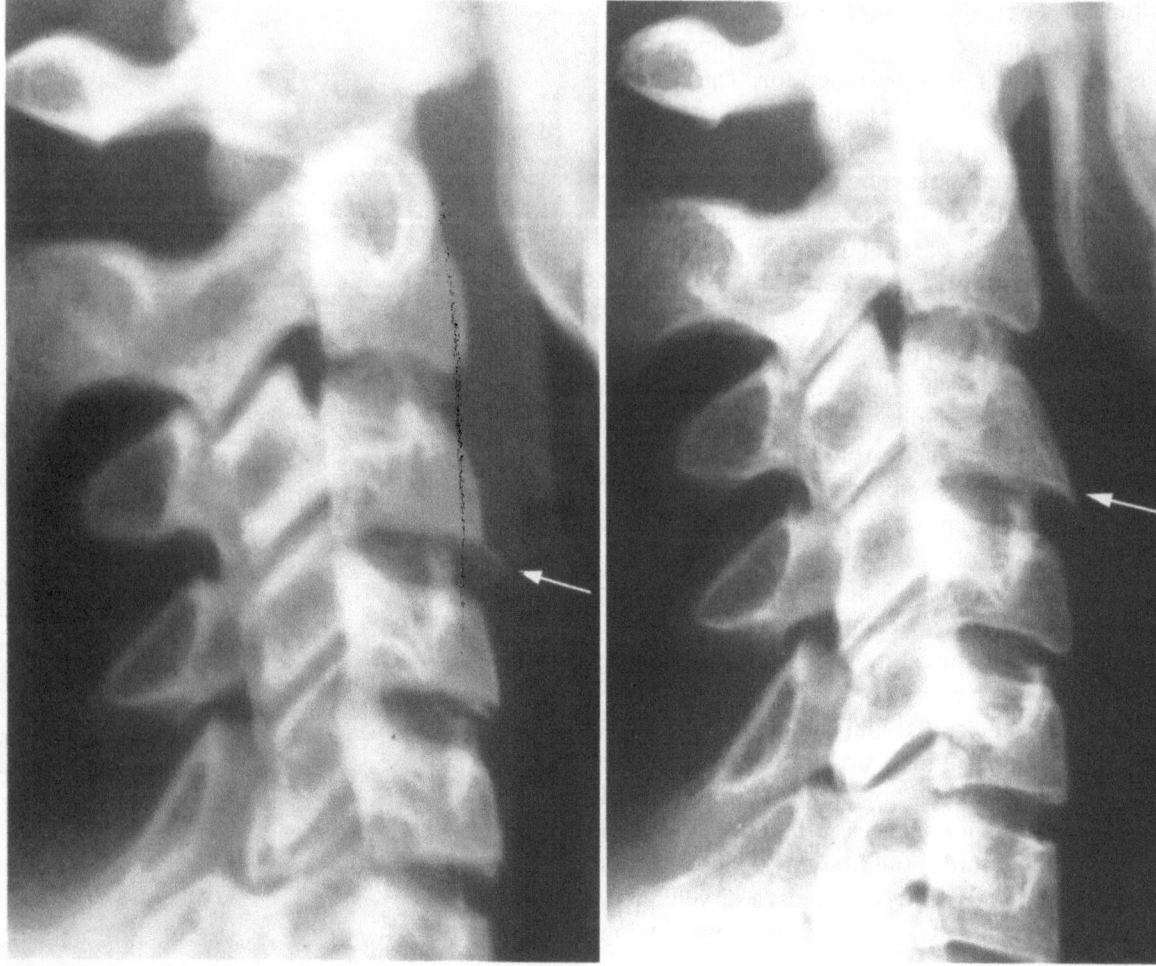

Fig. 41a, b. Anterior sprain. **a** Tearing-off of the annular epiphysis of C3 (→): anterior sprain. The hematoma that accompanies this traumatic lesion is seen as a swelling of the soft parts. On the X-ray picture taken 2 years later (**b**), note the deformation of the anterior wall of C3 (↦)

reveal segmental hypermobility such as that described above.

γ) *Anterior Sprain* (Figs. 40–42)

An anterior sprain is seen on a film taken in the extension position as an elective anterior intercorporeal widening (Figs. 40–42).

It is a serious matter if a severe cervical sprain that ought to receive surgical treatment (posterior fixation in the absence of an anterior lesion) is overlooked, and it may also be difficult to put forward a diagnosis in the presence of segmental hypermobility. As a matter of fact, hypermobility can be seen in a normal case under certain circumstances, and it would then be wrong to let a traumatized patient undergo aggressive therapy.

Angular kyphosis and segmental hypermobility can accompany the following conditions:

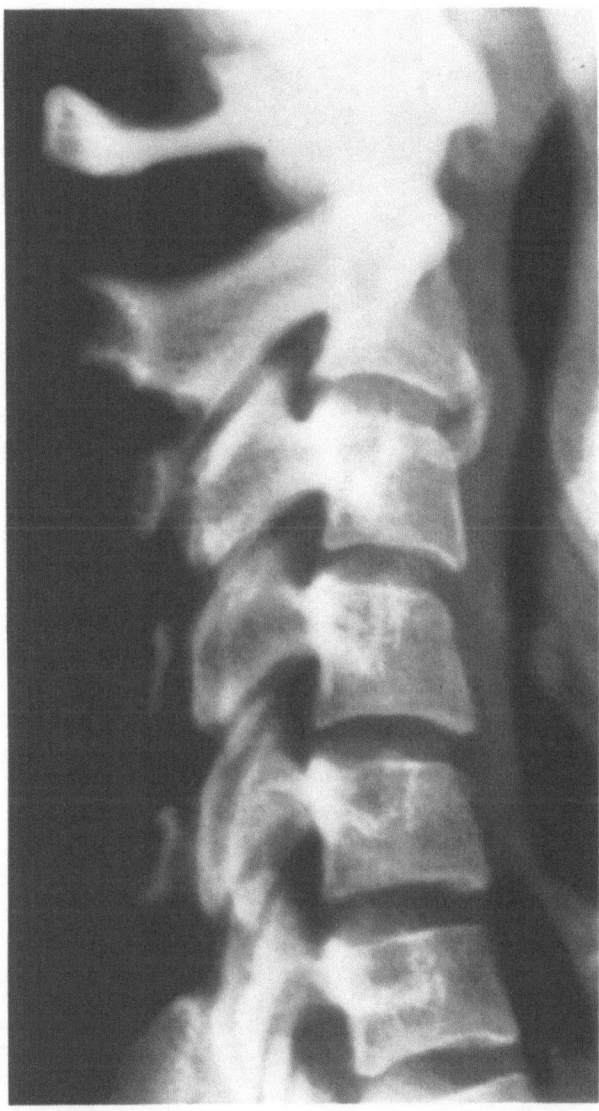

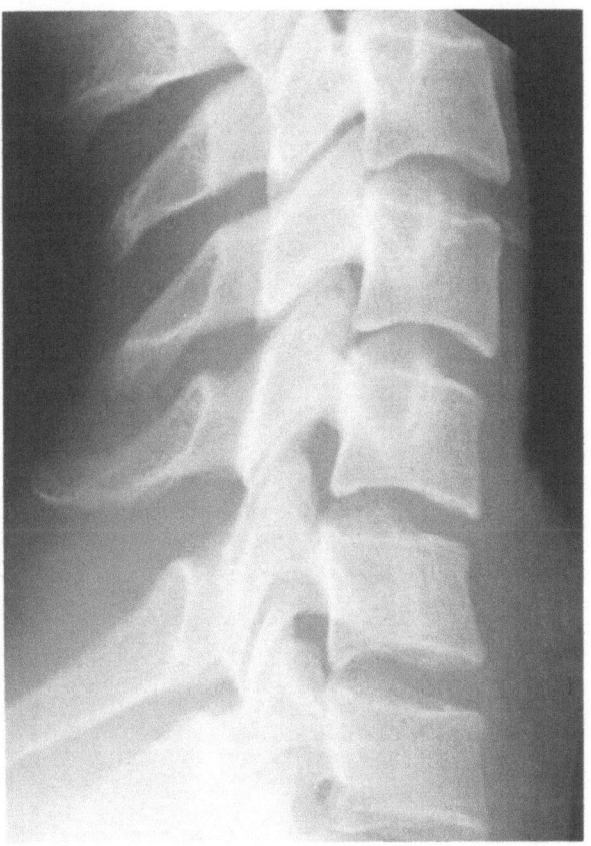

Fig. 42b. Severe posterior sprain (see text)

Fig. 42a. Anterior disk herniation with vacuolization and ossification of the anterior longitudinal ligament. This lesion had been overlooked 2 years previously, when the patient was X-rayed for a craniofacial trauma

Pre-existent arthritis of the disk: hypermobility is then only secondary to a pre-existent arthritic functional block at the level below.

A spine shaped like a figure 3 is usually the repercussion at the upper level of a flat back.

Localized hypertrophy of the posterior articular pillars due to a disturbance in the embryologic development.

In such conditions the clinical investigation takes on its full importance, and variants of normal are recorded when there is no elective interspinous painful spot at the level of the suspected sprain. It is then advisable to check these radiographic features later by means of dynamic studies. If the clinical examination does reveal the presence of an elective painful spot at the same level as the radiologic anomaly the sprain is diagnosed and adequately treated.

Chapter 3   Traumas of the Thoracic and Lumbar Spine

The thoracolumbar spine, and more specially the thoracolumbar joint, is the most frequent site of involvement in vertebral traumas. In contrast to the cervical spine, radiologic investigations and diagnosis do not present problems in this segment. Bone lesions are more frequent here than disco-ligamentous involvement. Pure luxations are exceptional and sprains are usually overlooked since they have no particular clinical and radiologic characteristics.

A. Radiologic Investigation Techniques

I. Conventional Roentgenograms

The radiologic investigations should be adapted to the individual patient's clinical state. In the case of neurologic damage (paraplegia, paraparesis, spinal cord syndrome, etc.) the initial investigation, as for the cervical segment, should comprise only a frontal and a lateral view, performed while the patient is lying on the stretcher and sometimes even through the molded mattress. These films are usually of very poor quality because of the abnormal magnification and because of inconvenient superimpositions, but they reveal any severe and unstable vertebral lesions and also provide some indication as to the steps to be taken when moving the injured patient onto the radiographic table. Thereupon the radiologic investigation is continued as for injuries without neurologic damage or minor traumas.

1. Thoracic Spine

Two orthogonal projections (a lateral and a frontal) are usually sufficient for a study of the vertebral bodies and the posterior arches. We use large-size films and do not focus too closely. Moreover, we take care to obtain a perfect superimposition of the vertebral end-plates so as to visualize the disk spaces. Therefore we recommend taking films with each incidence, one centered on the upper and the other on the lower thoracic spine. In case of doubt we perform a complementary incidence centered on the suspected spinal segment.

Because of the orientation of the posterior articular processes and of the laminae, oblique projections are not required unless a lesion of the posterior wall is suspected. This lesion is searched for on the vertebral body in the area between the two pedicles. Oblique projections are useful for the upper thoracic spine between C7 and T1, however, where a lateral view is not informative because of the superimposition of the shoulders. Under these conditions lateral tomograms should be routinely performed, as should a lateral view with high voltage; this may prove helpful taken with shifted shoulders.

2. Lumbar Spine

Besides the fundamental lateral and frontal projections, oblique projections are required when searching for fractures of the pars interarticularis. For the lumbosacral joint centered frontal, lateral, and oblique projections are compulsory.

II. Tomographic Investigation

We believe that tomograms are essential in the following circumstances:
1) Neurologic damage without obvious vertebral lesions
2) Vertebral fractures with marked displacement
3) Fruitless or insufficient vertebral reduction
4) Secondary displacement of a vertebra following a perfect reduction
5) Indication for surgery

In our daily practice we routinely perform to-mograms in all cases with neurologic damage and in all cases without neurologic damage but with severe bone involvements. This attitude helps, especially in the thoracic spine, to avoid overlooking lesions of the posterior arch, which are usually difficult to diagnose at this level, especially on the lateral film because the posterior costal arches are superimposed.

The patient must be positioned on a foam-rubber mattress, especially when there are signs of neurologic damage. Care must be taken to avoid pressure sores which could develop at the points of contact. Moreover, the patient must be immobilized, especially for the lateral tomograms to prevent shearing movements, which are eminently neuroaggressive. The tomographic investigation must include several vertebral levels and not only one or two vertebrae. For this investigation too, we use large-size films and usually a complex multidirectional tomographic movement.

B. Elementary Radiosemiology

We shall study lesions of the vertebral body and of the posterior arch in turn.

The classification of vertebral lesions is different in the thoracic and in the lumbar spine. However, they involve predominantly the thoracolumbar joint, which is a transitional area from both the anatomical and the functional point of view.

I. Body Lesions

Theoretically we distinguish fracture lines and vertebral compressions.

1. Fractures

The fracture line is a rupture in the continuity, which is seen on the film as a hypertranslucency on either side of which the bone structures, in particular the bone trabeculation, remain uninvolved.

The margins and the end-plates of the vertebrae usually remain rectilinear, and after reduction the vertebra resumes its normal anatomy. The orientation of the fracture line varies: it can be horizontal, vertical or oblique, and the displacements produced vary accordingly (Figs. 43–46).

a) Vertical Fracture Line

α) Frontal Type

This type of vertical fracture line extends from the upper end-plate to the lower in a frontal plane, and separates the vertebral body into an anterior part and a posterior part. The anterior part can be displaced forward and the posterior part backward, producing an increase in the AP diameters of the body. The backward displacement of the posterior wall is accompanied by a reduced AP diameter of the canal and may thus cause neurologic damage. In this mechanism the posterior arch is usually intact, which gives these lesions a stable appearance (Fig. 47).

β) Sagittal Type

In this type the fracture line extends from the upper plate to the lower plate in a sagittal plane; it separates the vertebra into a right and a left part. In case of interfractural diastasis the transverse diameter of the vertebra is increased; this is reflected in the interpedicular distance. Apertue of the anterior arch is usually associated with aperture of the posterior arch, and in these circumstances the latter is always injured. A careful analysis of the standard projections and of the tomograms almost always reveals the existence of a vertical fracture line, usually located at the level of the laminae. Unlike the previous type this one enlarges the intraspinal canal diameter, so that there is no cord compression.

b) Horizontal Fracture Line

The horizontal fracture line (Fig. 48) extends from the spinous process to the anterior vertebral edge and passes through the laminae, the articular pillars, and the pedicles. It separates the vertebra into an upper and a lower part. When the displacement is marked, as with luxations, distraction of the spinal cord and/or the nerve roots occurs, which may lead to definitive neurologic damage caused by rupture (paraplegia, cauda equina syndrome, etc.).

c) Oblique and Transverse Fracture Lines

In this category (Fig. 46) we classify all other types of fracture lines. These can be divided into elementary vertical and horizontal components according

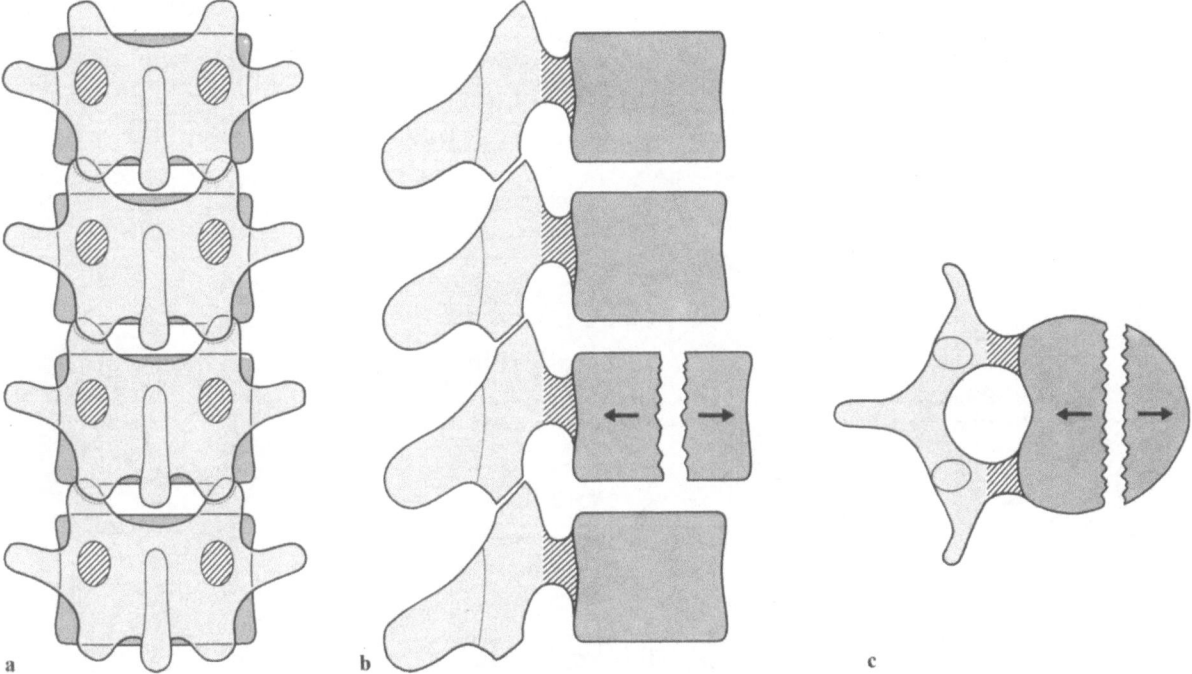

Fig. 43a–c. Vertical frontal fracture, frontal **(a)**, lateral **(b)**, and axial **(c)** views

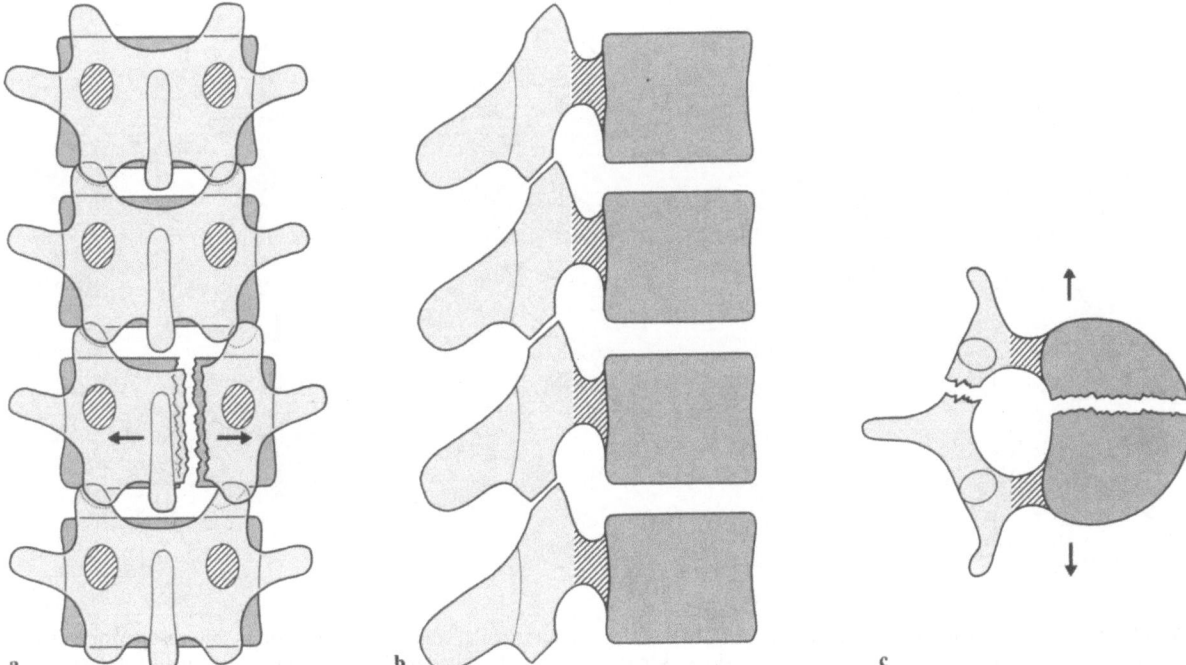

Fig. 44a–c. Vertical sagittal fracture, frontal **(a)** lateral **(b)**, and axial **(c)** views

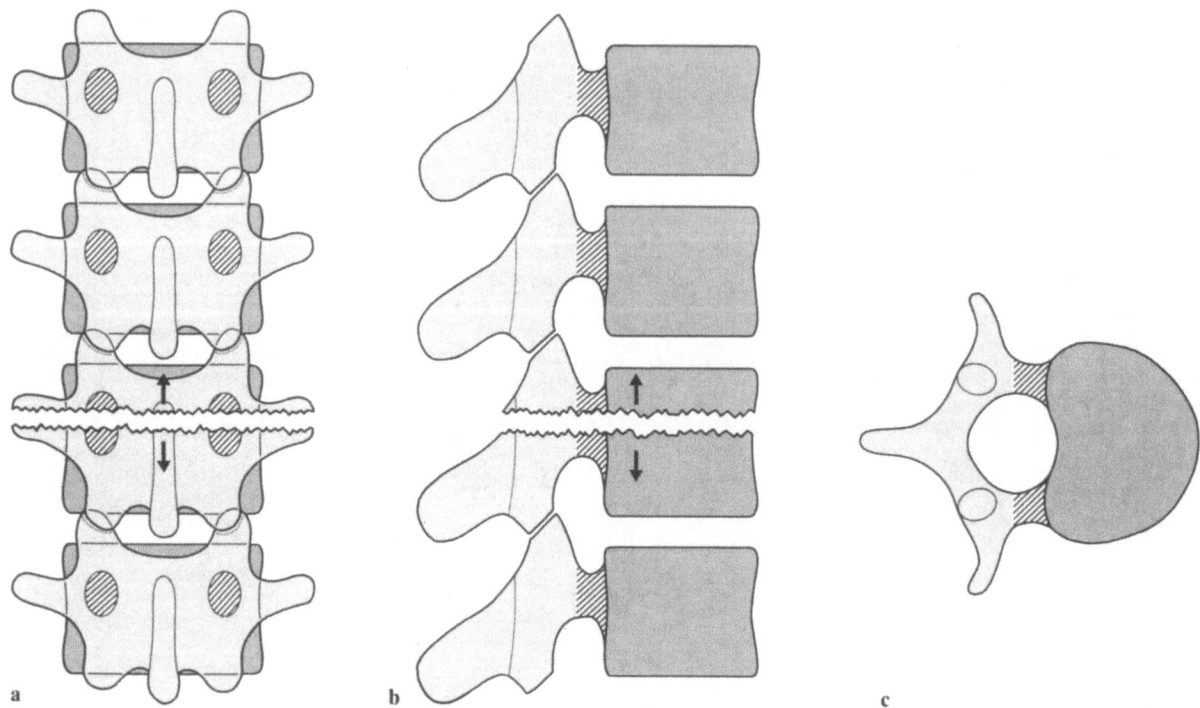

Fig. 45 a–c. Horizontal fracture, frontal **(a)** lateral **(b)**, and axial **(c)** views

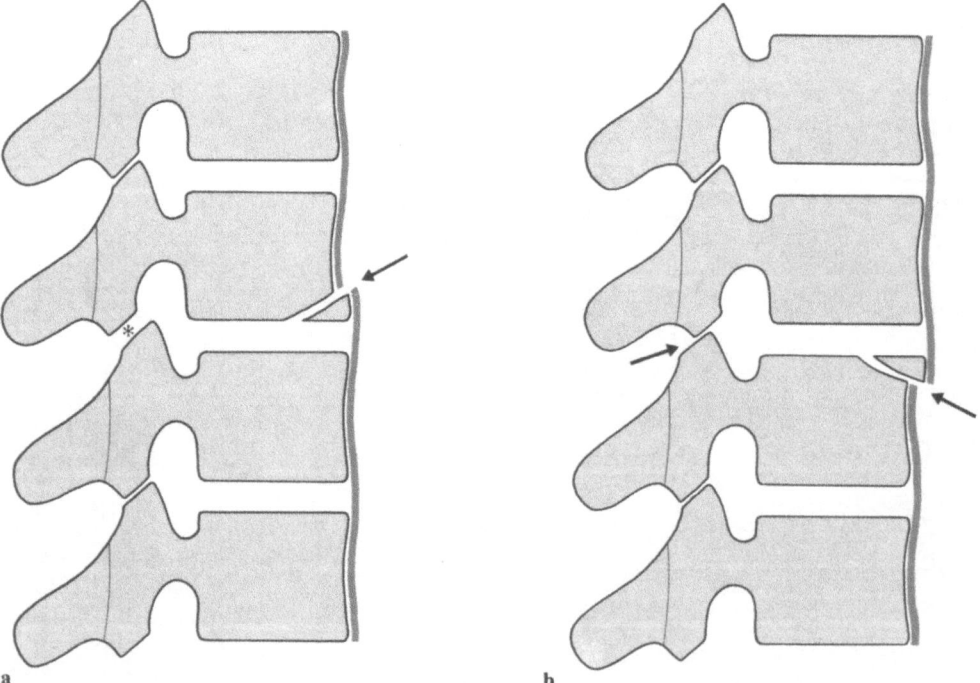

Fig. 46 a, b. Correlation between the involvement of the mobile spinal segment and the anterior vertebral bone lesions. **a** teardrop fracture: anteroinferior vertebral corner detached in the posterior direction with vertebral retrolisthesis and posterior interarticular diastasis; **b** luxation: anterosuperior vertebral corner detached in the anterior direction with antelisthesis and interarticular luxation

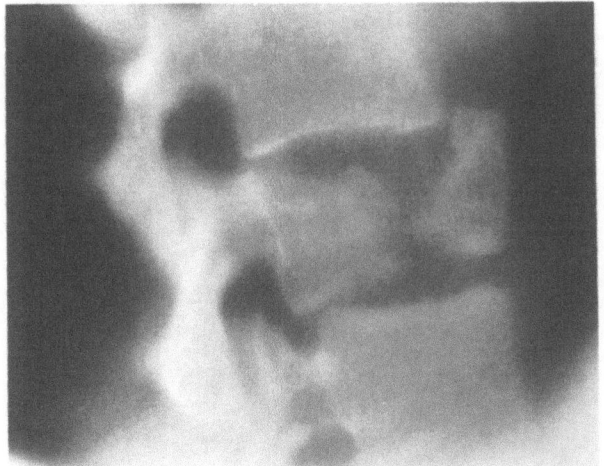

Fig. 47. Frontal vertical fracture of the L3 body. The patient landed flat on his back after falling from the first floor. No neurologic signs were present. The fracture line divides the vertebral into an anterior and a posterior part. The anterior part moves downward and the posterior part backward as a result of the posterior interarticular diastasis. The anterior and posterior walls are reduced but identical in height

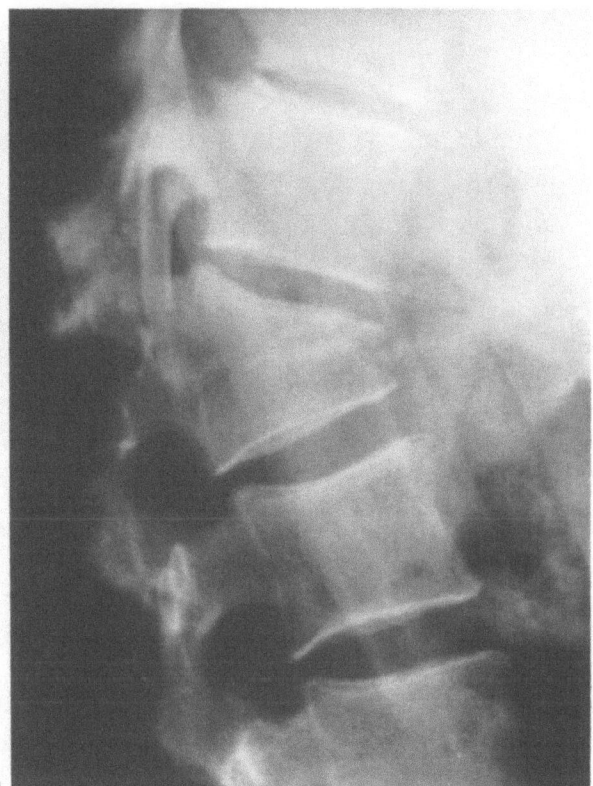

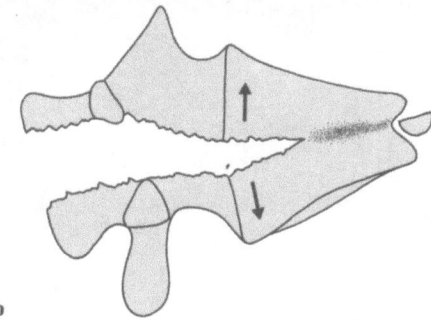

Fig. 48a, b. Seat-belt fracture: lesion by distraction. The horizontal fracture line divides the vertebra into an upper and a lower part. Note the increased height of the posterior wall relative to the adjacent vertebrae, in contrast to the compression of the anterior part of the body. In this type of lesion the means of union usually remain intact. Normal connections remain between the posterior interapophyseal joints above and below. The size of the intervertebral foramina is unchanged. **a** Lateral view. **b** Schematic representation

to the vectorial construction. Oblique fractures are located in the sagittal plane, transverse fracture lines in the frontal plane.

a) Oblique Fracture Line

Downward and Forward Oblique Fracture Lines. We distinguish three main types of these: oblique and short with no involvement of the posterior wall; oblique and of medium length, reaching the posterior wall on either side of the pedicles; and oblique and long, radiating to the posterior arch via the pedicles, which are thus injured as in lesions with horizontal fracture lines.

In this type of lesion one must always suspect involvement of the mobile spinal segment, i.e., ligamentous instability. Such an involvement is more likely to exist when the fracture line is oblique and short, in extreme cases causing avulsion of the anterosuperior corner of the vertebra, e.g., in the case of an intervertebral luxation. It is less likely when the fracture line is long, or, in the most extreme case, nonexistent, as in a horizontal fracture. This correlation is complemented by the notion of instability, as shown in Fig. 46. These fracture lines are usually oblique downward and forward, and are due to hyperflexion mechanisms.

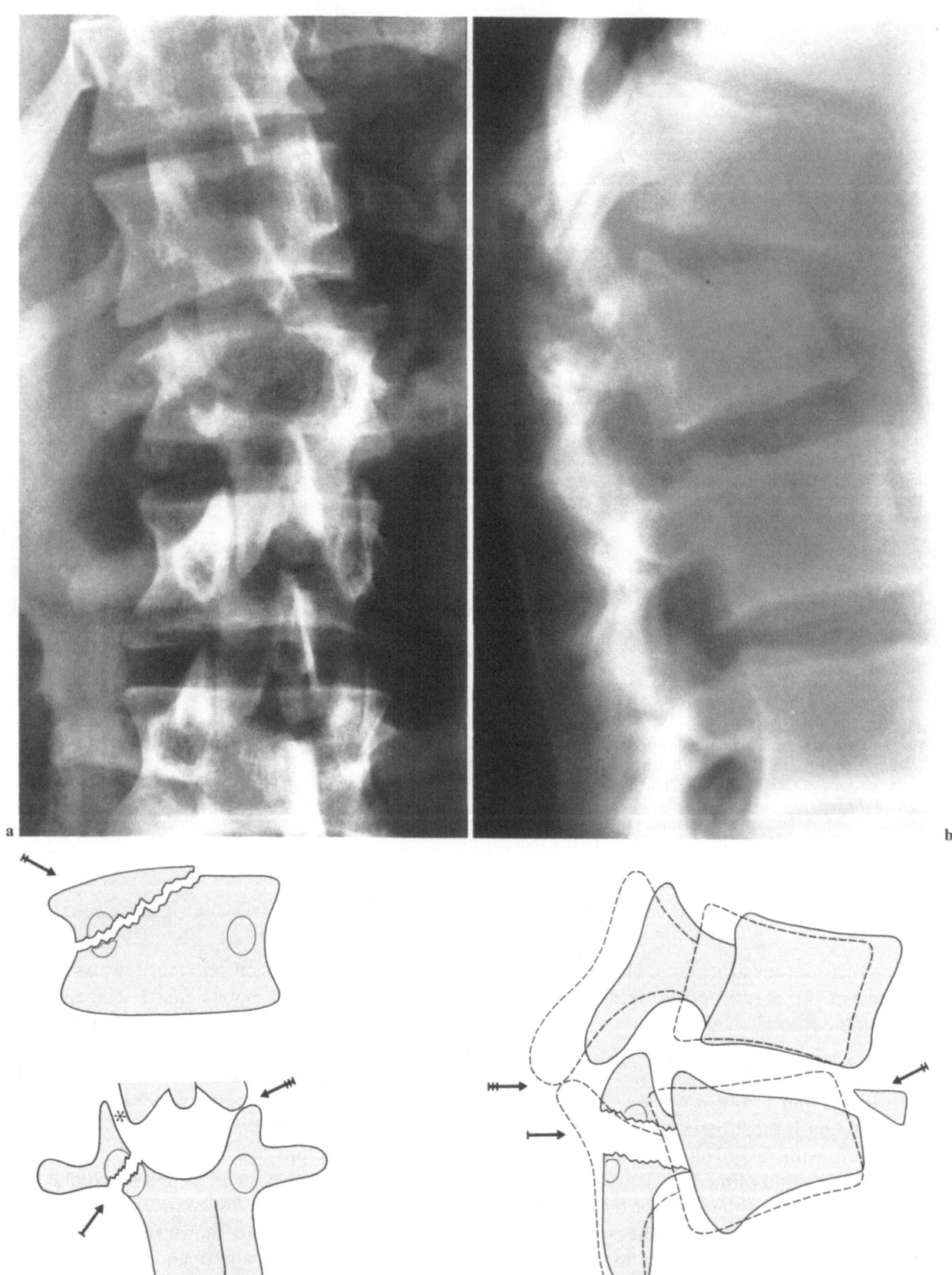

Fig. 49 a–c

Downward and Backward Oblique Fracture Lines.
A particular case is depicted in Fig. 65, with a
downward and backward fracture line. In almost
all cases these features are synonymous with
lesions secondary to hyperextension (tear-drop II)
or to inverted compression (tear-drop I).

β) Transverse Fracture Lines

Transverse fracture lines (Figs. 49 and 50) are
easily recognizable on frontal projections: they
extend from the vertebral plate to one of the lateral
aspects. Lesions of the posterior arch are con-
stantly associated and the fractures are located on a
line that is parallel to the fracture line of the body.
A lesion of this kind results from a shearing
mechanism.

2. Vertebral Compression

Vertebral compression is a lesion of the vertebra
without evidence of interruption in the continuity
but with an alteration in the bone trabeculation,
which becomes more dense and more opaque in the
injured part. There are changes in the contours of
the vertebra which tend to become convex or
concave. After reduction, in contrast to recovery in
the case of a lesion with a fracture line, the
anatomical restitution is never perfect and an
intrasomatic vacuum persists. This vacuum is
responsible for an iatrogenic, therapeutic, bony
and temporary instability. Thus, even after a well
conducted orthopedic treatment a residual compression remains.

   As for the fracture lines, different types of
vertebral compression can be described, i.e., partial corporeal compression (anterior, median, posterior, and lateral), and total corporeal compression.

a) Partial Corporeal Compression

Anterior or wedge compression (Fig. 51) is the
most frequent; it corresponds to compression of
the bone trabeculation of the anterior wall, which is

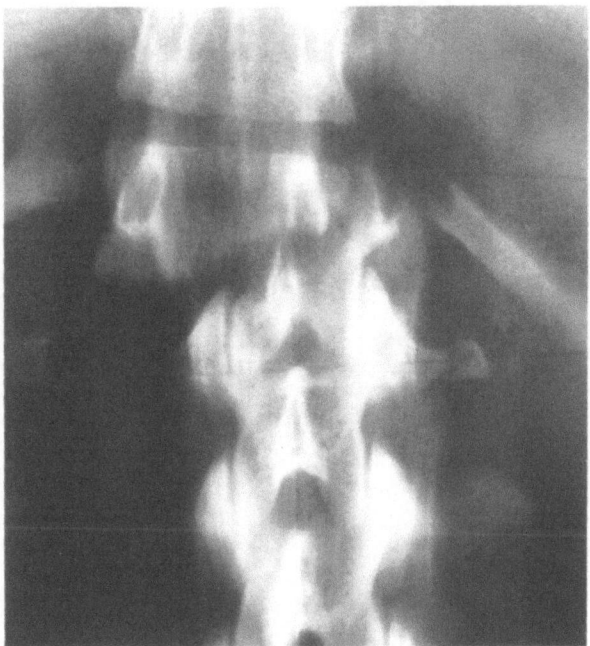

Fig. 50. Fracture of T12 by transverse shearing. Same direction
of anterior transverse fracture of the vertebral body and posterior lesions arch

an area of lesser resistance. It is usually caused by
forces of average significance acting on the spine in
flexion.

   The lesion can be minimal, and the following
radiologic signs should be looked for:

Densification of the anterior third of the vertebral
   body with moderate asymmetry of the anterior
   and posterior edges
Buckling of the anterosuperior part of the vertebral
   plate
Plication on the anterior aspect of the vertebral
   body

Medial Compression. The anterior and posterior
   walls are not involved; the lesions correspond to
   impaction of the nucleus pulposus into the adjacent vertebral end plate, usually the upper plate
   of the underlying vertebra.

◁ **Fig. 49 a–c.** T12-L1 transverse dislocation sustained in a street
accident during which the passenger had been ejected. No
neurologic signs were found. The lesions due to lateroflexion
are as follows (c):
On the *right* (side of the lateroflexion): fracture of the superior
articular process of L1, radiating to the pedicle (↦); fracture

disinsertion of the laterosuperior corner of the L1 body (↦);
transverse-type posterior interarticular disjunction (*); and
transverse fracture of the body.
On the *left* (posterior interarticular luxation; (⊪) the mechanism of the lesion accounts for the low importance of the
antelisthesis

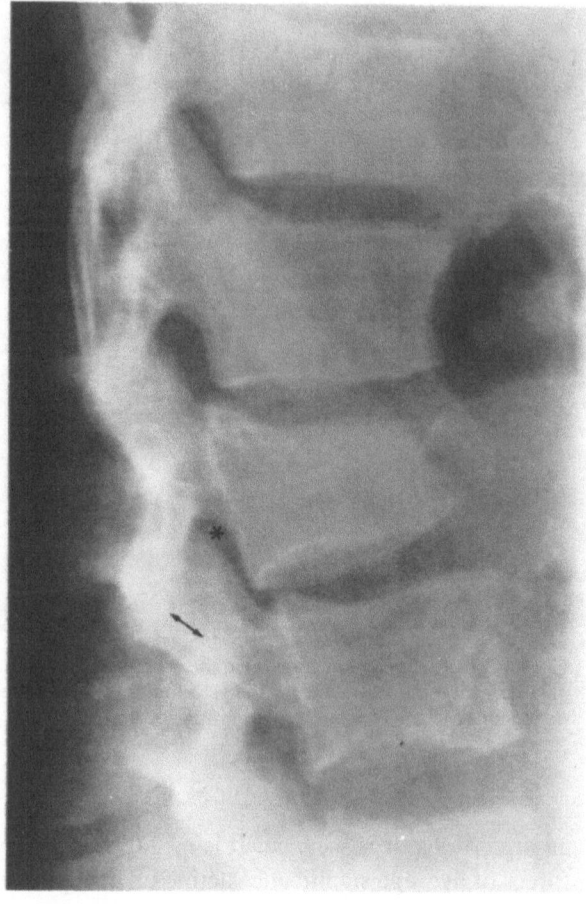

Fig. 51. Fracture by compression of the L2 body. Radicular pain of L2 type was reported. The lateral view reveals anterior wedge compression with intact posterior wall. Retrolisthesis of L2 relative to L3 is responsible for a global backward displacement of the posterior wall associated with enlarged ($\leftrightarrow$), posterior articular L2–L3 space, resulting in the reduced projection area of the L2–L3 (*) intervertebral canal, which explains the radicular pains

Fig. 52a, b. Global corporeal compression of L2, standard $\triangleright$ (a) and tomographic (b) lateral views. Disinsertion of the anterior wall with a frontal vertical fracture line is seen. Vertebral compression predominates in the central part. Backward displacement of the superior part of the posterior wall into the vertebral canal ($\mapsto$). Marked widening of the posterior articular L2–L3 interspace, indicating concomitant backward move of the posterior arch (*)

Such a lesion can be caused by landing flat on the back after a fall. Because of the anatomical predisposition it is then located at the level of the thoracolumbar joint.

Posterior compression is exceptional. When such a lesion does occur it is always seen on an abnormal vertebra, in which the posterior wall has been weakened either by a tumoral or by a dysplastic process.

Lateral compression is visualized on a frontal projection. It resuls from an injury in lateroflexion or in rotation. When it occurs in children or young adults it can lead to scoliotic disturbances in the axial static.

In these different types of compression the posterior wall is usually not involved, so that they are not neurotoxic. This is not the case for the lesion described below.

b) Total Corporeal Compression

Like partial compression, total compression (Fig. 52) results from an axial compression force. If this force is applied to an erect spine the compression is symmetrical, i.e., equal on the anterior and posterior aspects. When the force is applied on a flexed spine the compression in the anterior part of the body is predominant. These features are easily recognized on the radiographs: in symmetrical total compression the adjacent vertebral plates of the intact vertebrae remain parallel, while in asymmetrical total compression the same end-plates show angular kyphosis of variable degree.

There is also enlargement of all diameters of the injured body, and particularly of the AP diameter, with protrusion of a part of the posterior wall into the spinal canal. The backward shift of the posterior wall causes more damage when the posterior arch remains intact.

This is fortunately rare.

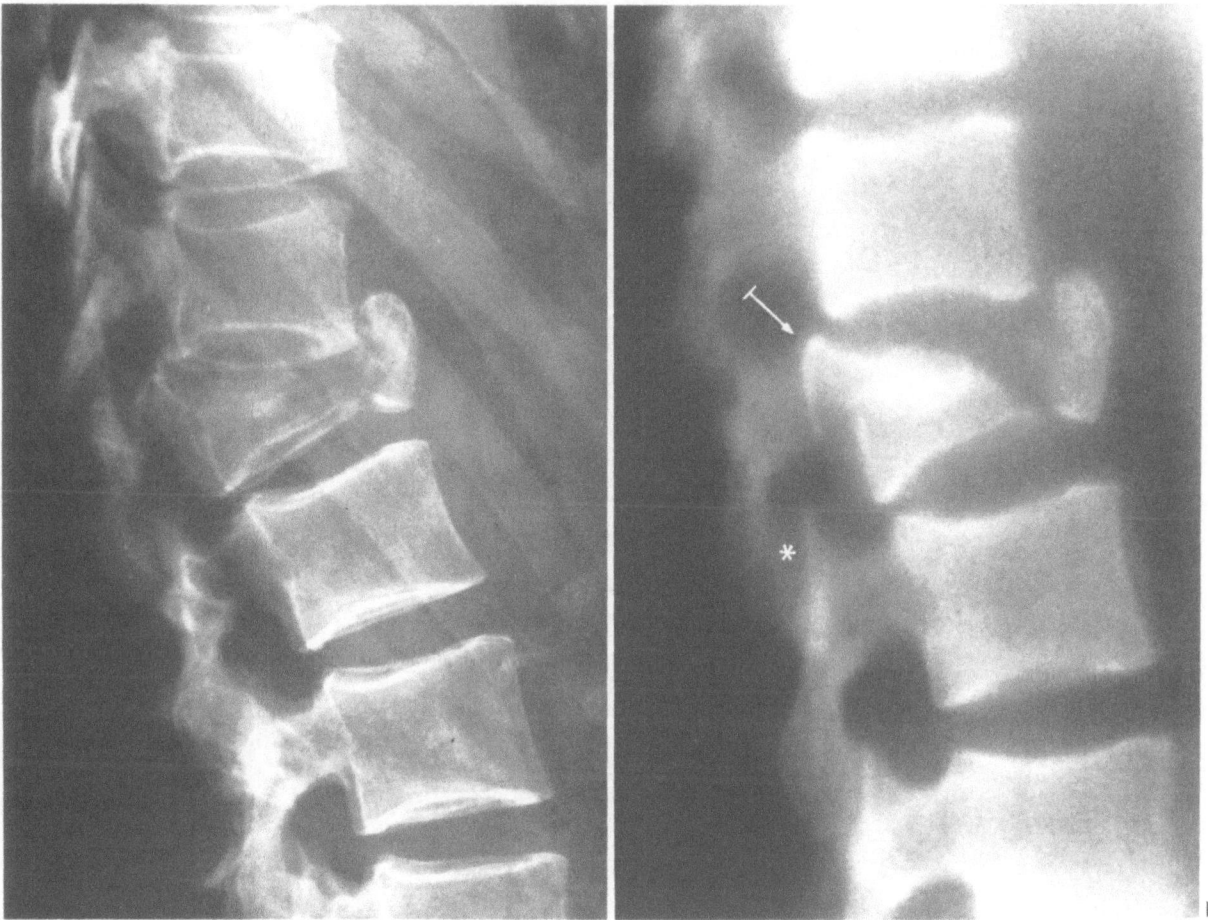

Fig. 52a, b

II. Lesions of the Posterior Arch

1. Isolated Lesions

Isolated lesions of the posterior arch (Fig. 53), for instance of the articular processes, are exceptional compared with those occurring in the cervical spine, but are frequently associated with corporeal lesions. Fractures of the "accessory" spinous and transverse processes are more frequent.

Fractures of the *spinous processes* occur either on the occasion of a direct blow or, more probably, during hyperextension or hyperflexion movements. In hyperextension, the lesion results from impaction between two adjacent spinous processes. In hyperflexion it is the result of traction forces. The fracture line then has two orientations, depending on the level of the lesion on the mobile spinal segment. For the vertebra below, the fracture line runs obliquely downward and forward.

For the vertebra above, it is oblique in an upward and forward direction. Thus the direction of the fracture line shows which mobile spinal segment has been injured.

The *transverse processes* provide insertion for the greater psoas muscle. Fractures at this level are secondary either to excessive traction — in which case they are often symmetrical — or to excessive rotation, when they are asymmetrical.

2. Associated with Body Lesions

Any fracture, any compression of a vertebral body should lead to carefully search for one or several concomittant lesions of the posterior arch.

The tomographic investigation permits an excellent analysis and reveals three fundamental types of fracture lines: vertical, horizontal or oblique.

These types of lesions can be pure or mixed, uni or bilateral, symmetrical or asymmetrical.

A
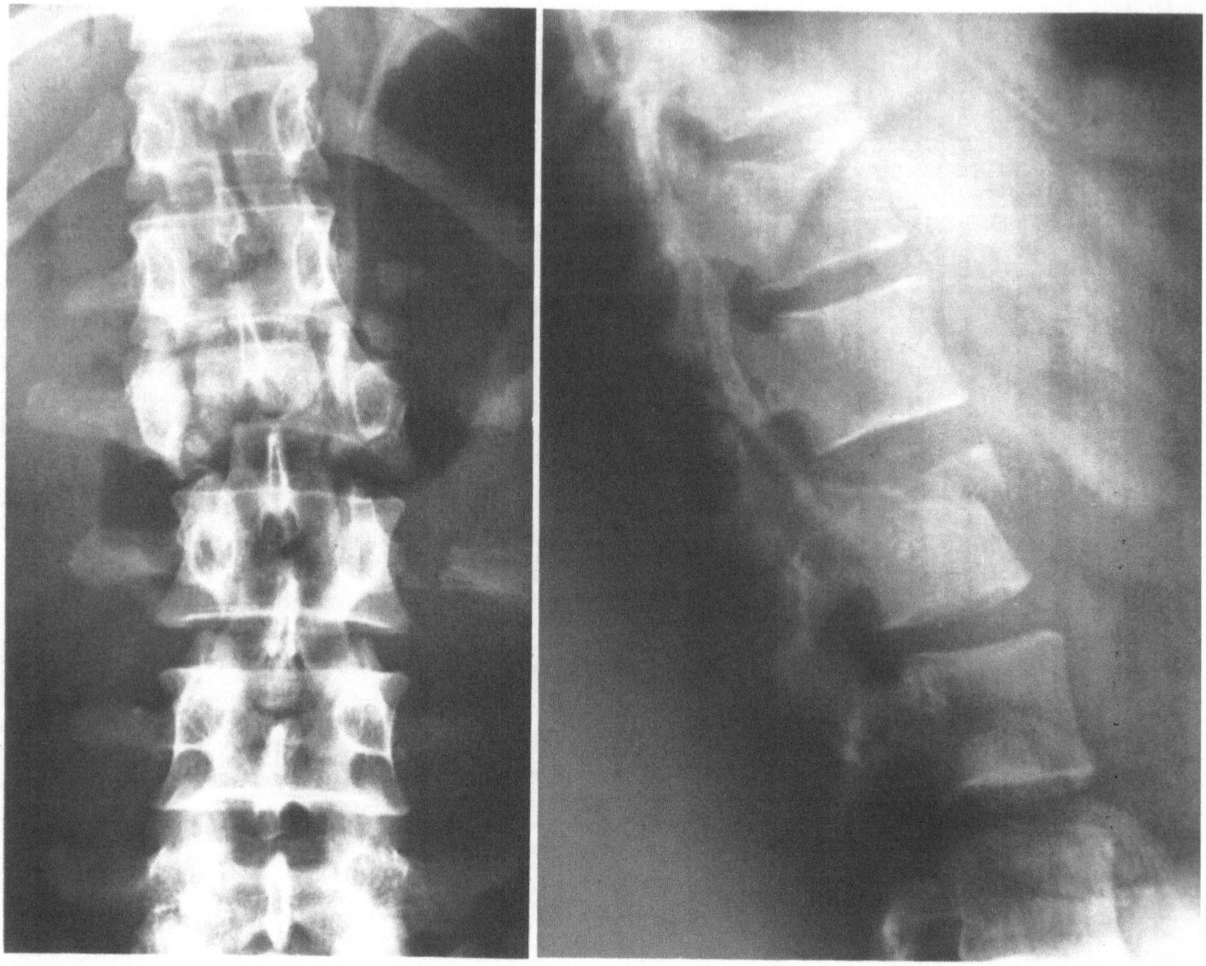
a b

Fig. 53 A–C. Multivertebral lesions in a patient who fell from a height of 20 meters. Complete paraplegia, level T12.
A Standard projections.
B Frontal tomogram showing the lesions of the posterior arches of L1 **(a)** and of L2 **(b)** (→). Note the predominance of isthmic fractures (→) and the marked right posterior interarticular L1–2 dislocation (*).
C Lateral tomogram on large-size films showing the severity of the thoracic lesions that the standard films had failed to demonstrate. Multiple fracture of the superior articular processes with luxation T11–T10 (↦), isthmic fracture of L1 (⇸), and fracture of spinous processes (○→)

Their existence plays a fundamental role for the comprehension of the mechanism of the lesion; we believe indeed each type to reflect a given mechanism, namely:
— the vertically directed fractures result from a compression mechanism (Fig. 53).
— the horizontally directed fractures result from an avulsion mechanism (Fig. 48 and 57).
— obliquely directed fractures would be synonymous of a shearing mechanism (Fig. 50).

The coexistence of vertical and horizontal fractures is the sign of more complex fractures such as a fracture due to rotation with a lateral rotation axis (Fig. 70), associating, on the side of the pivot, a vertical fracture by compression, and on the opposite side, a horizontal fracture by distraction.

III. Luxations and Sprains

1. Isolated Lesions

Thoracic and lumbar luxations are not unusual (Fig. 54). They most often involve the thoracolum-

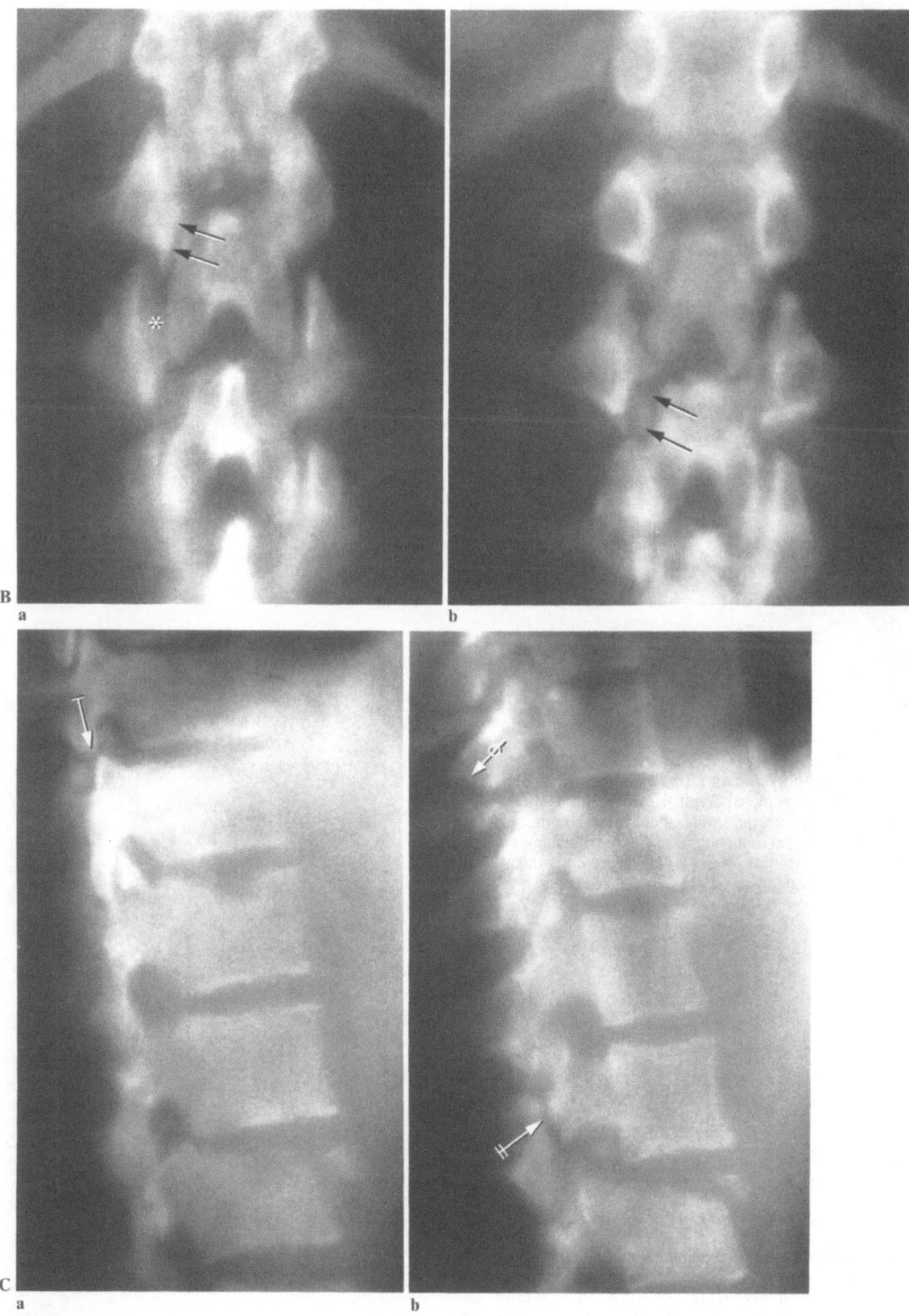

Fig. 53 B, C

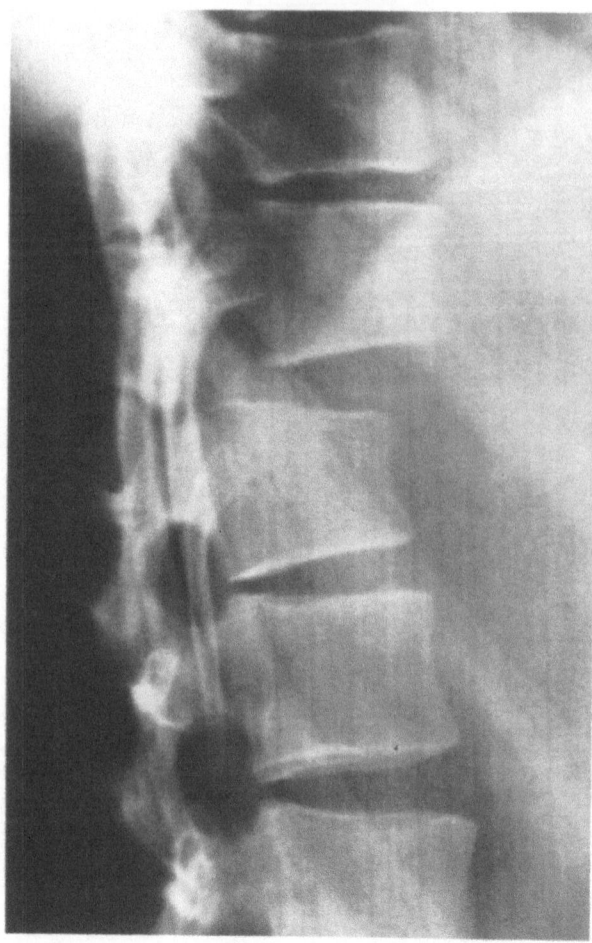

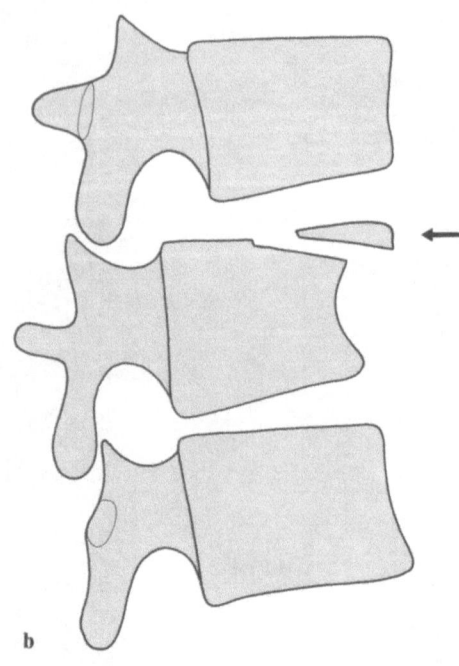

Fig. 54a, b. Luxation of T12 on L1 following a horse-riding accident, resulting in complete paraplegia with marked antelisthesis of T12 on L1 and posterior interapophyseal over the top luxation requiring surgical reduction. Disinsertion of the underlying anterior discovertebral plate (→) has occurred with the displacement of the luxated vertebra

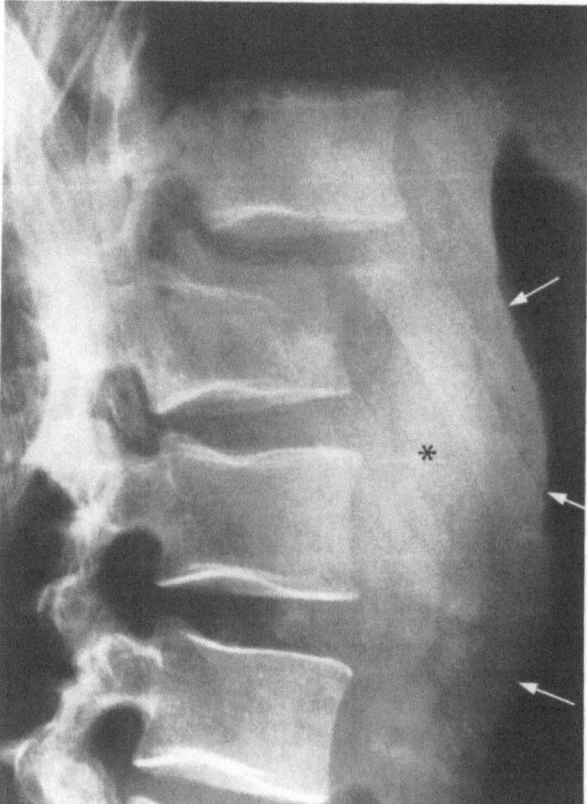

Fig. 55. T12–L1 luxation with median oblique fracture line of the vertebra below. The vertebral body fragment thus separated remains attached to the intervertebral disk and is concomitantly displaced. A marked hematoma (*) pushes the posterior aspect of the stomach forward (→)

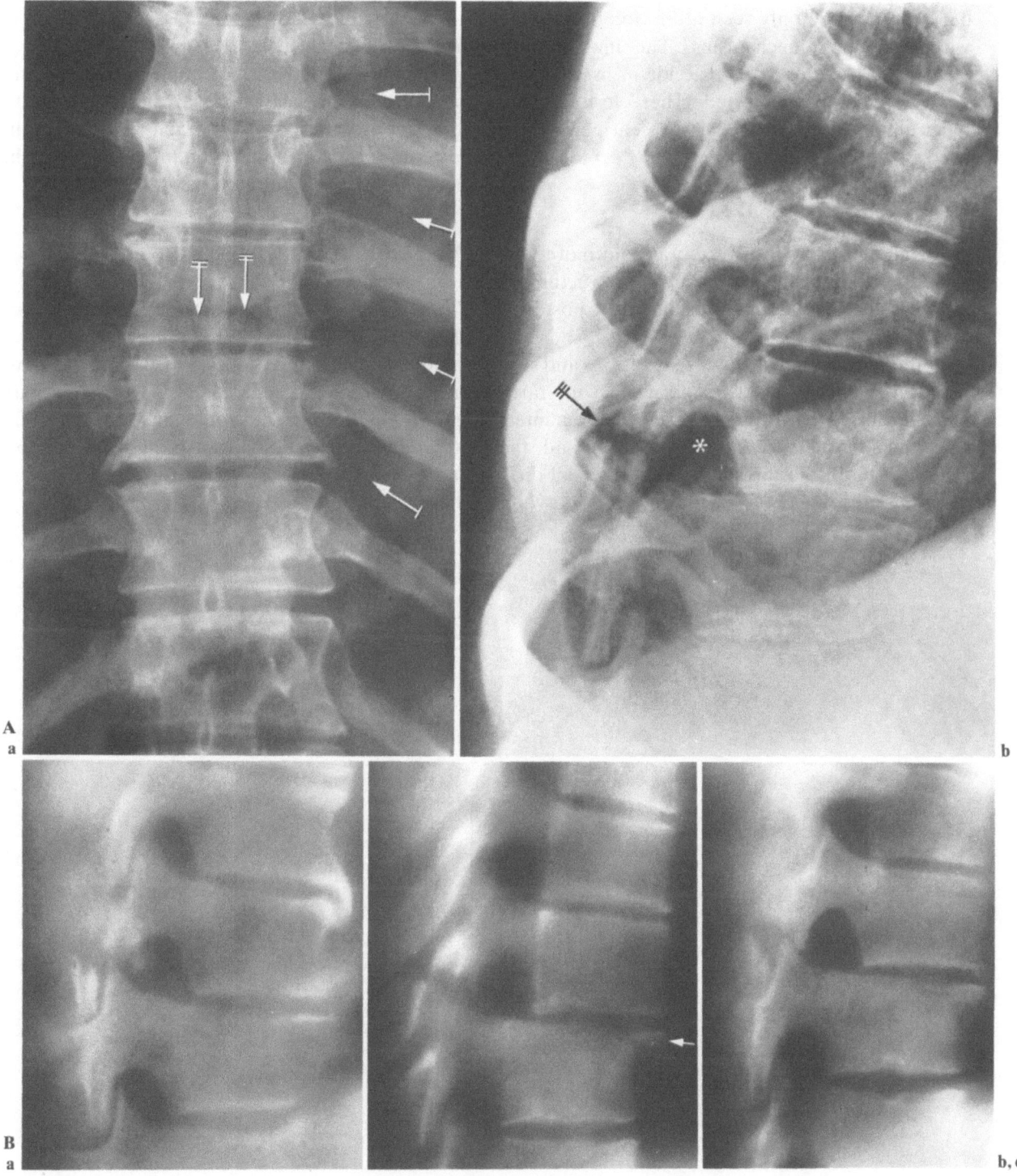

Fig. 56A, B. T8–T9 fracture luxation due to a shearing mechanism. The case concerns a patient with multiple traumas after a traffic accident. The initial radiographic investigation was incomplete. The back pain was said to be due to fractures of the ribs. The diagnosis was made 8 days later when a posterior cord syndrome was noted when the patient stood upright.

A The frontal projection (**a**) shows a marked (→) displacement of the left paravertebral alignment (→) and a rupture in the continuity in projection of the T9 body (⊦→). The lateral view (**b**) shows the luxation (⊪→). Note the hypervisibility of the intervertebral foramen (*).

B Tomograms. The lesions of the posterior arch involve the right (**a**) and left (**c**) inferior articular processes and the lamina (**b**) of the luxated T8 vertebra. Disinsertion of the anterosuperior corner of the below has occurred (→). The lesions are due to a shearing mechanism

bar joint and are only seen after violent traumas with distraction mechanisms. The most typical example is provided by road accidents in which the passenger has been ejected. These lesions were particularly frequent when lap seat-belts were used.

2. Associated with Body Lesions

Involvement of the intervertebral, and more particularly posterior interarticular joint structures is just as frequent as the bony lesions of the posterior arch.

Although we easily recognize luxations and subluxations we had a tendency to neglect interarticular diastases located in the axial plane, namely the transverse diastases (Fig. 53 Ba) and the anteroporterior diastases (Fig. 51). An axial diastasis must always be suspected in body lesions with ante or retrolisthesis, without associated lesion of the posterior arch.

When it is associated with anterior body lesions, the presence of such an axial diastasis permits, alike the orientation of the fractures lines on the posterior arch, a better comprehension of the mechanisms of traumatic vertebral lesions.

IV. Soft Parts

The study of the soft parts is helpful only in lesions of the thoracic spine. The radiograms show a spindle-shaped image consistent with a perivertebral hematoma (Figs. 55 and 56). This sign is particularly significant; it should always attract the attention of the radiologist, especially in comatose patients. It serves as a warning signal on a routine chest radiogram.

Chapter 4   Comprehensive Study

The elementary lesions of the spine described in Chapter 2 can occur in isolation or in combination. Once they have been diagnosed it is important to determine the prognosis of the lesions and to integrate them into a given classification.

A. Lesional Diagnosis

From the initial radioclinical investigation we retain three fundamental characters, i.e., rupture in the continuity, displacement, and the complications that can result from any trauma to the spine, whether this is direct or indirect in nature.

I. Rupture in the Continuity

When a rupture affects the bone structure it is a fracture or a compression. When it concerns the discoligamentous structures, we speak of a severe sprain or luxation; in the event of a luxation we note a complete rupture of the posterior ligamentous structures, and even involvement of the posterior longitudinal ligament in the case of bilateral luxation. In the case of unilateral luxation the posterior longitudinal ligament spared to a greater or lesser extent. With severe sprains rupture of the ligaments is not always complete, so that we prefer to speak of distension.

We shall consider later the prognosis of these two varieties of lesions. The genesis of rupture in the continuity remains unknown however. Why does it, under almost identical circumstances, involve either the vertebral bone or the means of union? Should the muscle tone be taken into account? The most striking example is constituted by contrasting bilateral luxation and seat-belt fracture (Figs. 57 and 58).

II. Displacements and Listhesis

The presence of listhesis should always suggest involvement of the posterior arch. Listhesis was long considered to be synonymous with luxation. In fact it can also be related to fracture displacement or interosseous diastasis. Usually tomography provides evidence of the cause of the listhesis. Although this distinction is artificial it seems to us important, and even paramount as far as the cervical spine is concerned.

As a matter of fact, in the case of purely interosseous diastasis in which the rupture in the continuity disinserts the upper articular process from the lower (i.e., fracture of the isthmic part; type III lateralized antelisthesis), there is no lesion of the posterior interarticular means of union between the vertebrae above and below. Reduction is usually easy and healing is obtained after bone consolidation.

Conversely, for types I, II, and IV lateralized antelisthesis, i.e., unilateral luxation, fracture of articular processes, and fracture-separation of the articular pillar, the lesions of the means of union are constant. Reduction of the antelisthesis can be difficult, sometimes even requiring surgery. Healing is only obtained after consolidation of the bone and discoligamentous lesions.

The exact extent of the displacement has no great significance in traumatic pathology. As a matter of fact the initial radiographic investigations never correspond to the patient's initial status at the time of the accident, and the amplitude of the movements that have caused the displacements will always remain unknown. Therefore the importance of the displacement seen on the initial radiographs is always minimized, and it remains underrated because of either spontaneous or manual reduction during transportation of the patient from the site of the accident to the X-ray department.

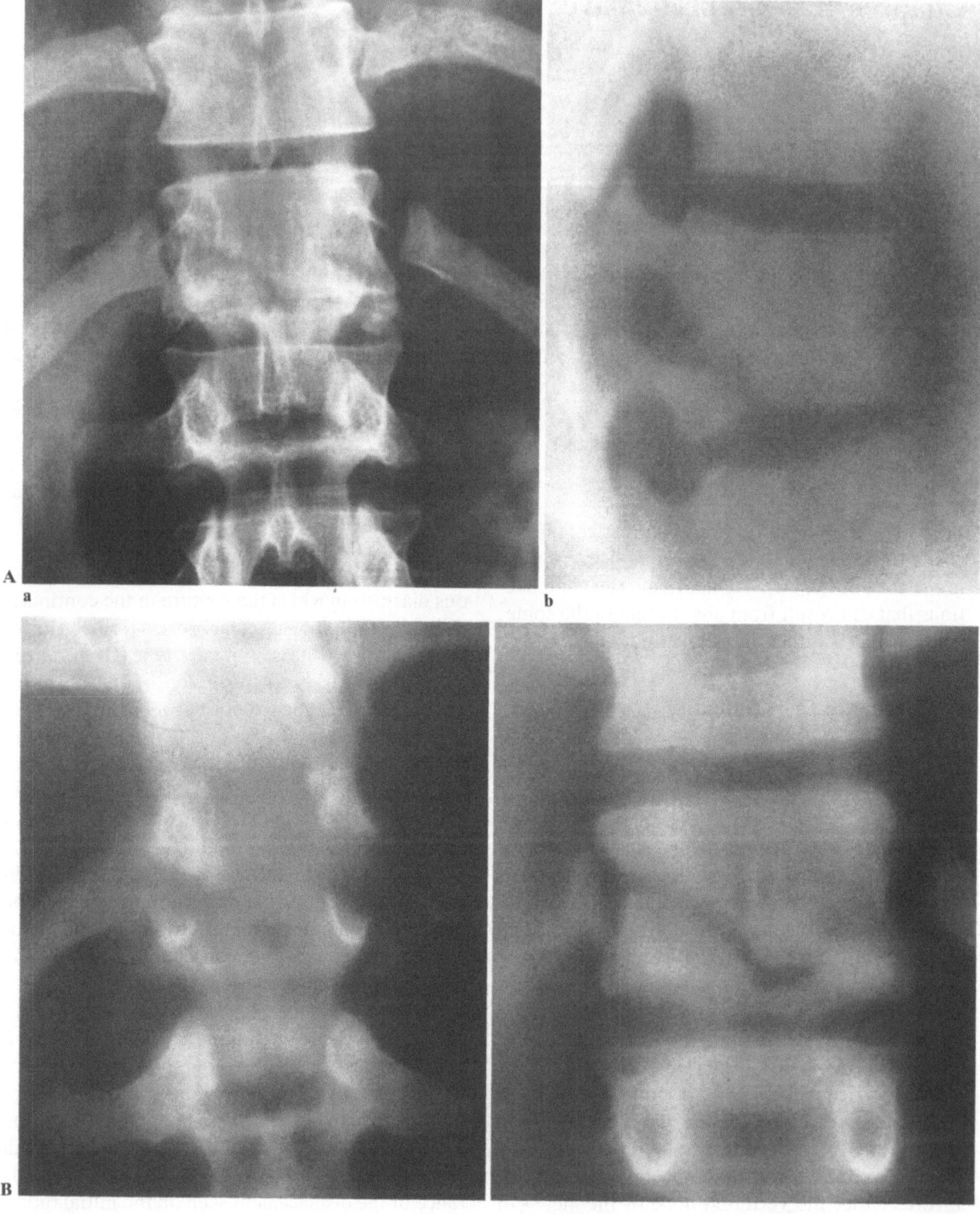

Fig. 57 A, B. Chance fracture of T12 (seat-belt fracture) sustained in a motorcycle accident. No neurologic signs are apparent. The fracture line is markedly oblique from above downward and from back to front; it involves the pedicles and terminates on the posteroinferior aspect of the end-plate.

A frontal **(a)** and lateral **(b)** standard view.
B frontal tomograms

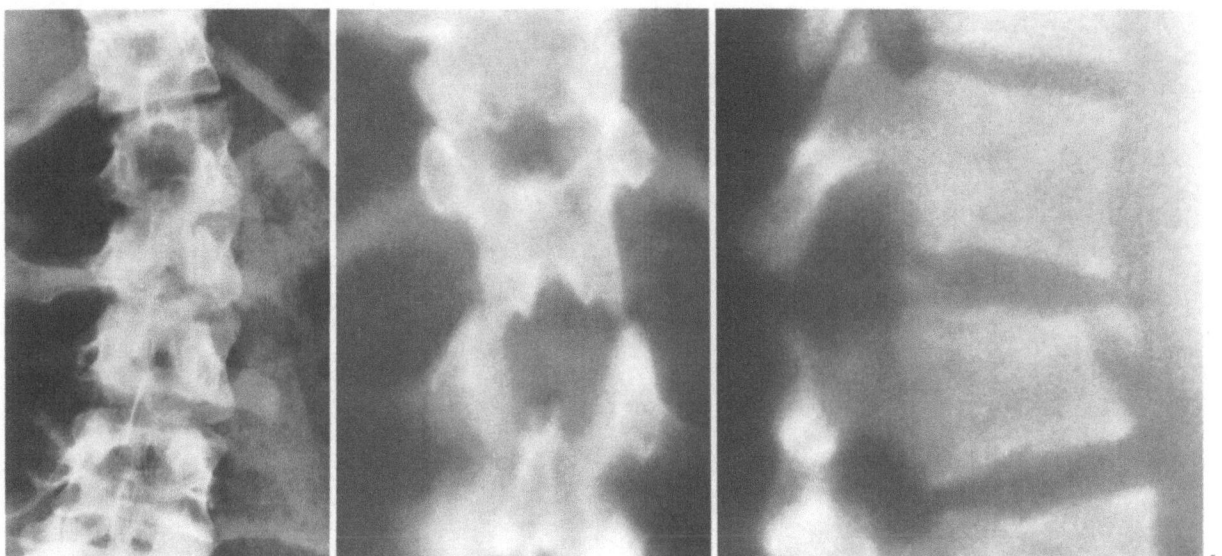

a   b, c

Fig. 58a–c. Luxation T12–L1 with widening of the interspinous space (**a, b**) and avulsion of posterior corner of T12 and of the anterior corner of L1 (**c**)

III. Vasculonervous Complications

1. Nervous Complications

The existence of a displacement is not necessarily synonymous with vasculonervous complications, and vice versa. A discrepance between the clinical and radiologic data is frequent, as is confirmed in daily practice. Displacements are nevertheless eminently toxic when they occur in cases with narrowness or stenosis, of a canal, whether acquired or congenital.

Depending on the clinical data, the radiologist performs the radiologic investigation as follows:

a) Traumatic Spine with Cord Compression Syndrome

With reference to the bones, the radiologist should search for lesions on the vertebral spinal canal margins, and especially for a lesion of the posterior wall; as far as the ligaments are concerned it is important not to overlook a spontaneously reduced luxation. As evidence of this we look for tearing-off or avulsion of an anterosuperior corner of a vertebra associated with a hematoma of the prevertebral soft parts.

If neither of these two lesions is present a vascular cause (medullary ischemia following rupture or thrombosis of the anterior spinal axis), an enucleated disk, or even an extradural spinal hematoma should be considered.

Hence the importance of the positive-contrast investigations, which, however, are replaced by CT examinations in the more specialized departments. These have the advantage of allowing simultaneous study of the bone structures and of the intra- and extraspinal soft parts.

b) Traumatic Spine with Radicular Syndrome

In this case a lesion of the intervertebral foramen must be looked for: fracture of an articular process, fracture-separation of an articular pillar, or unilateral articular luxation. In the absence of a radiographically visualized lesion, further investigations are carried out to look for a lesion of the brachial plexus or a posterolateral disk herniation.

c) Traumatic Spine Without Neurologic Signs

This can occur in any of three situations:
Isolated, benign, and usually stable bone lesions that do not require surgery
Bone and ligamentous lesions that are obviously progressive. In this case severe complications might occur because of secondary displacement, for example:

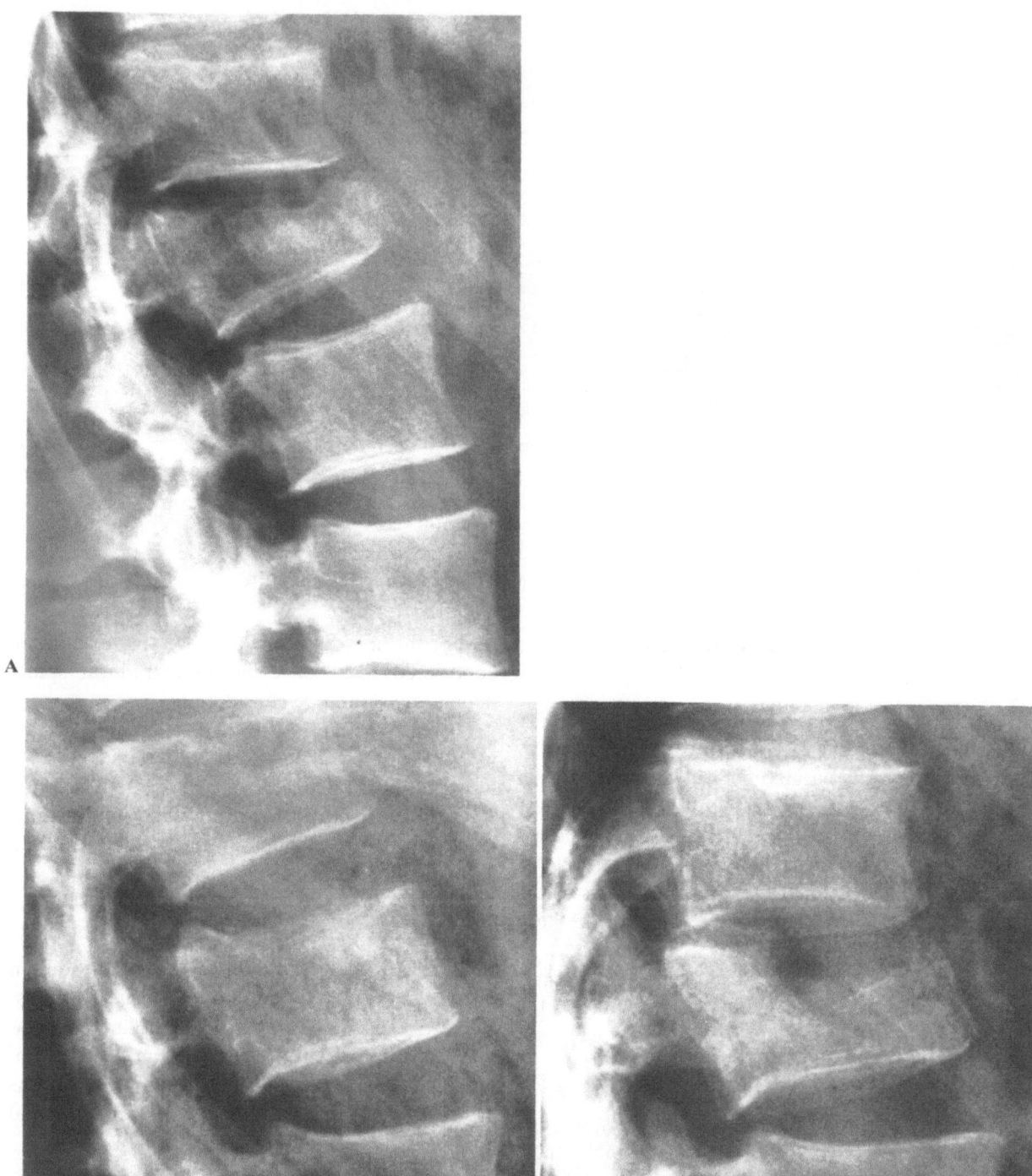

Fig. 59 A, B. Global compression with backward displacement of the posterior wall, showing initial lesion (**A**) and status following orthopedic treatment (**B**) with perfect restitution of the height of the vertebral body after reduction (**a**) and occurrence of a secondary compression, indicating the bony instability of the lesion (**b**)

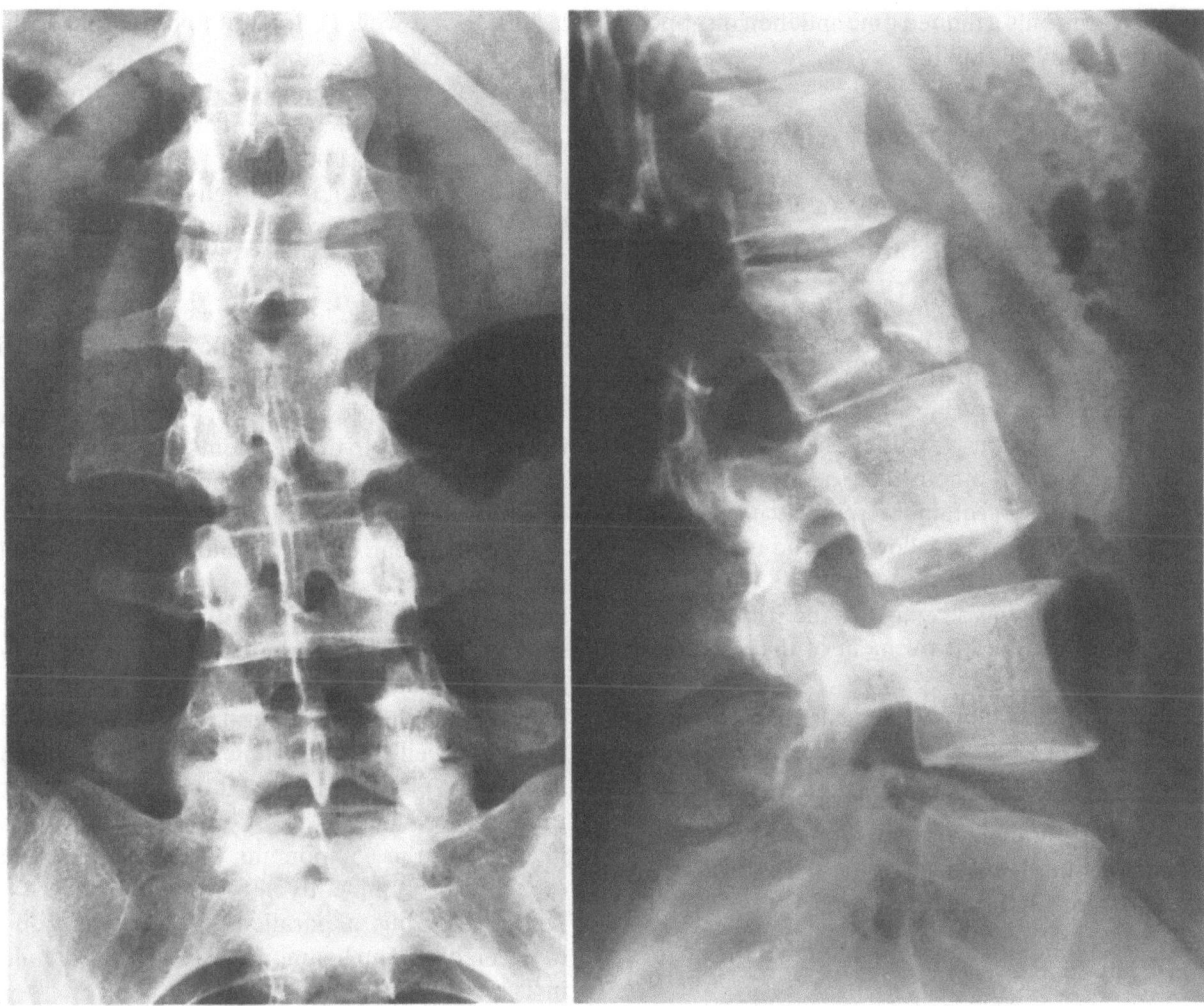

Fig. 60. Frontal vertical fracture of L2, associated with a mediocorporeal compression. The lesion was found 3 weeks after an accident, in the absence of neurologic signs. This shows the good stability of this type of lesion, but there is a risk of pseudarthrosis

Fracture of the odontoid with an obliquely downward and backward fracture line
Type II fracture of the axis pedicles
Body fracture extending to the posterior wall
Involvement of the transverse ligament

Absence of any bone lesion. This leads automatically to institution of a search for a severe sprain

2. Vascular Complications

The involvement of cephalad vessels, e. g., vertebral and carotid arteries, is exceptional. Various publications report arterial thrombosis and intramural hematomas. In our daily practice the lesion most often encountered is carotid artery dissection, occurring in cases with craniofacial traumatism in hyperextension.

B. Dynamic Functional Diagnosis

Once a vertebral lesion has been recognized it is necessary to assess the prognosis, with particular reference to its stability or instability. A lesion is said to be *stable* when no secondary displacement has occurred spontaneously or following reduction. It is called *unstable* if under the same conditions it has caused a secondary displacement. The instability is durable to a greater or lesser extent, and we distinguish between temporary instability, which lasts only a limited time and then disappears, and definitive instability.

I. Bony Instability (Figs. 59 and 60)

Pure bone lesions are usually stable or temporarily unstable. As LOUIS (LOUIS 1977, LOUIS and GOUTALLIER 1977) has stated, the instability results mainly from involvement of the columns (anterior pillar and posterior articular column) rather than from the bridging and means of union (pedicles laminae) (Figs. 59 und 60).

Isolated lesions to the accessory processes (transverse and spinous) are usually negligible.

For the thoracolumbar spine LOUIS proposes rating the lesions as follows for the assessment of instability:

1 point for the involvement of the columns
0.5 point for the involvement of the pedicles and laminae
0.25 point for the involvement of the accessory processes

With 2 points or more there is very likely to be instability, and from 3 points or more bony instability is definitely present.

II. Discoligamentous Instability (Fig. 61)

Except for benign sprains, the discoligamentous lesions (Fig. 61) are definitely unstable. For these lesions too, it would be useful to establish a rating scale, as for bone instability:

1 point for lesions of the disk, the posterior and the anterior longitudinal ligament, and the posterior interarticular ligament
0.5 point for a lesion of the ligamentum flavum
0.25 point for a lesion of the intersupraspinous and intertransverse ligaments.

Below 2 points, the instability is minor and corresponds to a benign sprain, while above 3 points it is always definitive. There is however an exception. Unlike the bony lesions, which can be found in isolation, lesions to the ligaments are always associated with others, and one cannot conceive of a lesion to the posterior longitudinal ligament without involvement of the elements of the mobile spinal segment in front or behind it. Therefore all lesions of the posterior longitudinal ligament are evidenced by a severe sprain and instability on the dynamic studies.

For example, a unilateral luxation is usually stable and well tolerated clinically, which is why the diagnosis is often made late, at the arthritic stage of the disease, whereas a tear-drop fracture, which involves all the components of the mobile spinal segment, is prominently neuroaggressive.

There is thus a parallelism of the instability between bony and ligamentous lesions, as detailed in Table 3.

While the bony lesions are easy to recognize, the ligamentous ones raise many diagnostic problems.

Table 3. Correlation between bone and discoligamentous instability

	Anterior column			Bridge	Posterior column	Bridge	Accessory processes	
Bone	Anterior wall	Body	Posterior wall	Pedicle	Articular pillars	Lamina	Spinous	Transverse
Ligaments	Anterior longitudinal ligament	Disk	Posterior longitudinal ligament		Ligaments and inter-articular capsules	Ligamentum flavum	Inter-supraspinous ligament	Inter-transverse ligament
Quotation		1		0.5	1	0.5	0.25	0.25
					Spinal canal			
Clinical equivalent of purely ligamentous lesions	Anterior sprain					Benign posterior sprain		
	Tear-drop fracture type II					Severe posterior sprain		
					Luxation			

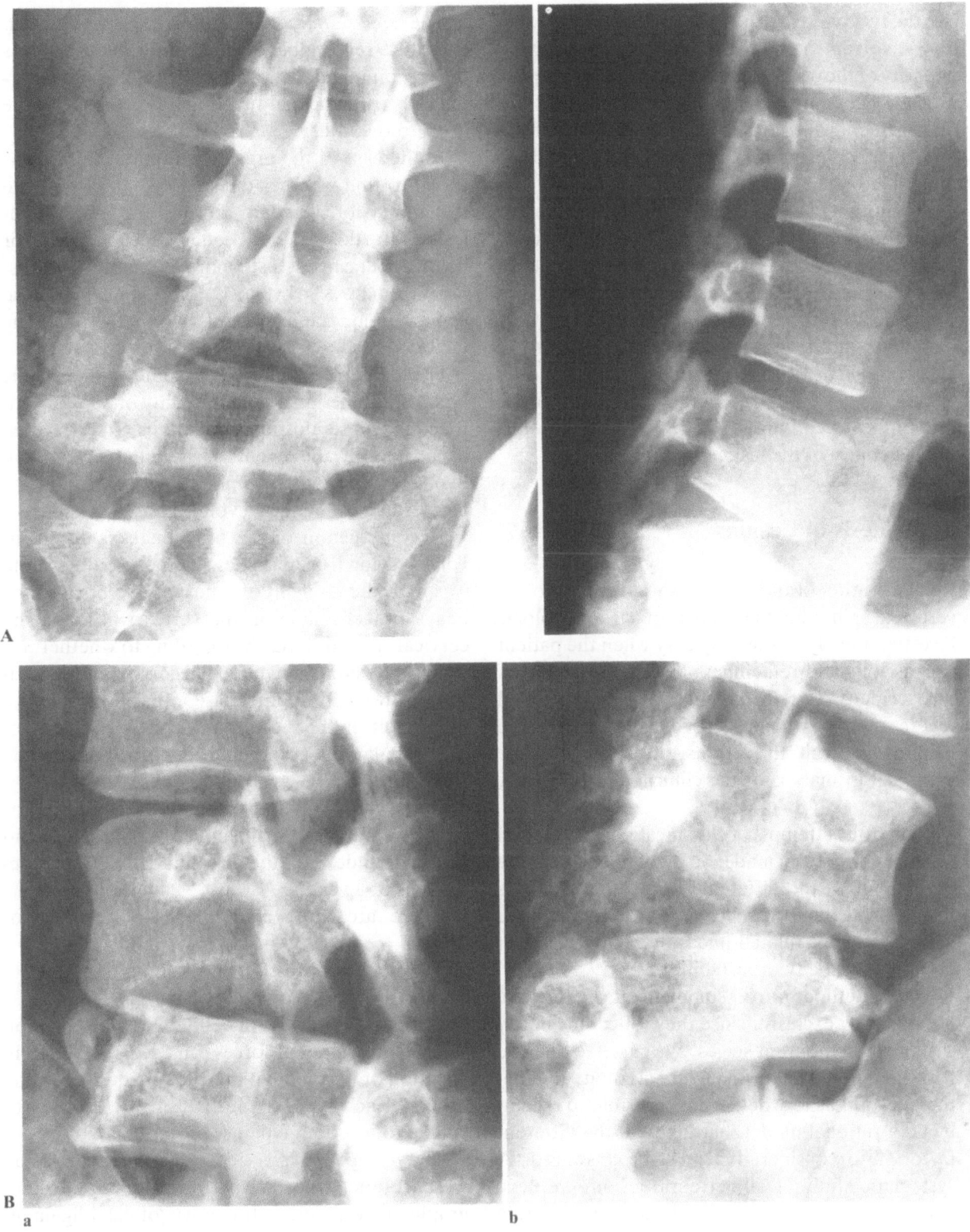

Fig. 61 A, B. Severe sprain L4–L5, which has led to L4–L5 luxation within 6 months in spite of orthopedic treatment. **A** frontal and lateral view taken with the patient upright; sciatica on right; walking was possible the help of crutches;

B right (**a**) and left (**b**) posterior oblique projection. The initial radiograms had been performed in India following a traffic accident. They show radiologic signs of severe sprain identical with those in Fig. 64

But the two types of lesion are also often contradictory, involvement of one sort of tissue ensuring the integrity of the other. Thus a fracture of the spinous processes guarantees the integrity of the interspinous ligament, and conversely, involvement of the interspinous ligament is a sure indication of bone integrity.

This notion of a definitive instability of lesions to the mobile spinal segment is fundamental as far as mixed lesions, whose potential evolution depends on the severity of the ligamentous lesions, are concerned. If these are severe the instability is definitive, and if they are minor it is temporary. The coefficient of total instability is obtained by adding up the coefficients of bony and ligamentous instabilities according to Table 3. Above 3 points the instability of the lesion is major.

C. Genesis of Lesions

Reconstitution of the mechanisms of injury to the vertebral spine should be a part of a traumatologic investigation. This is usually easy when the patient is conscious and remembers the circumstances of the accident. But in patients with multiple and severe traumas, who have lost consciousness or are unable to recall the events, the only possible approach is analysis of the clinical and radiologic signs.

Numerous attempts at classification of vertebral fractures have been made. Some of them are based on analysis of the different fracture lines; others take into account the mechanisms; still others are more treatment related and only take account of notions of stability or instability.

These methods are all complementary; they are not mutually exclusive since they reflect the injury sustained, at different stages. We curselves believe that they should all be taken into account, and that the question as to whether it is possible to recommend a rational model that takes all the different factors into consideration must be answered. A systematic study of all vertebral lesions we have encountered permits an overall and more occurate view, in the absence of a perfect synthesis.

Examination of an injury to the spine comprises three stages, i.e., pre-, per-, and postlesional stages.

The *prelesional stage* is often neglected, which can cause regrettable errors in interpretation. It is thus recommanded that attempts be made to determine the organic and functional state of the spine prior to the injury.

In the case of the organic condition, this means trying to find whether the spine was intact before the injury or whether there were pre-existent lesions (arthrosis, functional blocks above or below, metastases, osteoporosis, malformations, SCHEUERMANN's kyphosis, etc.), in which case even a minor trauma would be only the revealing factor.

For example, an arthritic spine with organic block and functional hypermobility or suprajacent reactional pseudospondylolisthesis can become dislocated in the event of a minor trauma in hyperflexion (Fig. 36). In this case the trauma has accelerated the natural evolution of the lesion.

Reconstruction of the functional condition involves trying to determine what position the spine was in at the moment of injury. Quite obviously a heavy object falling on the vertex will affect the cervical spine differently according to whether it is in hyperflexion, in hyperextension, or in the neutral position. In the first case a tear-drop fracture may result, in the second, a fracture-dislocation of the articular pillar, and in the third, a JEFFERSON's fracture.

In the *lesional stage*, trauma acts as a force for which we must define the direction, the sense, and the magnitude, i.e., the three fundamental characteristics of a vector.

There are three main planes of exertion of forces:
a) vertical: compression and distraction
b) horizontal: AP or lateral shearing
c) rotatory: clockwise or counterclockwise torsion

The three types of forces can each be exerted in isolation or in combination with one or both of the others. Each type of mechanism predisposes of course to a certain type of lesion.

The *postlesional stage* corresponds to the lesion we encounter when we perform the initial radiographic investigation. It consists of osteoligamentous lesions with or without displacement.

There is quite obviously a relationship between the cause and the effect for these different stages, but will the mere visualization of the effects allow recognition of their cause? On the basis of the following remarks we think that it is possible.

The direction of the fracture line corresponds to the direction of the force if this is exerted in isolation. If forces are exerted simultaneously in several directions the fracture line will be superposable on the resultant forces

The way in which the force is exerted is given by the direction of the initial displacements

The intensity is a physical magnitude depending on the energy released on the occasion of the trauma.

There are three main types of energy:

a) Kinetic energy: $E_c = 1/2\, mv^2$
   in frontal and lateral shocks

b) Potential energy: $E_P = 1/2\, mgh$
   in vertical falls

c) Kinetic moment: $E_M\ 1/2\, m\omega^2$
   for rotational forces

Any energy accumulated before the traumatic impact is quickly released and dissipates in all directions. Lesions occur as soon as the intensity of this energy exceeds the threshold intensity needed to rupture the different elements that constitute the vertebral column. For an equal energetic level, the lesions start at the points where the rupture threshold is lowest. This is a fundamental notion which makes it possible to understand why the same type of mechanism can cause entirely different lesions. At this stage the role of the dorsal muscle tone is a vital factor. For example, a blow applied in the upper thoracic region can cause, depending on the muscle tone, either a fracture due to a shearing movement at the point of application of the forces or a distant intervertebral luxation, usually in T12–L1.

We come here to a point of paramount significance in traumatology of the spine: there is no correlation between the circumstances of the accident and the nature of the lesions, and vice versa. The radiologic investigation remains fundamental to recognition of the type of the lesions, however.

In Chapter 5 the different types of lesions are considered with reference to the three main action planes of the forces.

Chapter 5   Classification

A. Lesions Caused by Distraction Forces

I. In Flexion

Such lesions always occur at the level of the posterior vertebral arch, either on the spinous processes or on the interspinous ligaments. The mechanism causes two types of lesions, depending on whether it involves the discoligamentous or the bony structures.

1. Discoligamentous Lesions

a) Luxation

The radiologic signs of such lesions are well known. In this case the posterior articular processes on either side of the mobile spinal segment remain intact (Fig. 62). On the posterior aspect, however, depending on the resistance of the interspinous ligament and on the tension of the posterior paravertebral muscular structures, the lesion can start at the level of the spinous process rather than the fracture line indicating the level of the injured spinal segment. It runs obliquely down- and forward for the vertebra above and obliquely up- and forward for the vertebra below. On the anterior aspect the sign of the luxation can be avulsion of the anterosuperior vertebral corner. In contrast there is never anterior wedge compression as in luxations due to compression on a flexed spine.

This distinction is of basic importance with regard to the study of the instability. As a matter of fact, in luxations by distraction the instability is always posterior, discoligamentous, durable, and definitive. In luxations due to compression-flexion, there is also anterior instability of bony origin (Fig. 63).

b) Sprain

Among traumas of the cervical and the lumbar spine we recognize severe and benign sprains (Fig. 64).

2. Bony Lesions (Seat-Belt Fracture; Fig. 48)

In its purest form, the horizontal fracture line passes through the spinous process, the laminae, the pars interarticularis, the transverse processes, the pedicles, and the body. It thus divides the vertebra into two hemivertebrae, a superior and an inferior part, which remain attached to the above and below lying vertebrae respectively.

Displacement is upward and forward, as in luxations, but the discoligamentous structures remain intact. Depending on the origin and on the end of the fracture line we recognize different forms. Thus the fracture line starts of the back at the level of the laminae or of the pars interarticularis after having ruptured the posterior ligamentous structures, and extends forward to the upper or lower vertebral plate. In any case the involvement is symmetrical in the sagittal plane.

If the involvements are asymmetrical a rotatory force must be suspected. In this event the distraction force is no longer centered on the median pivot represented by the nucleus pulposus, but on a lateral pivot. Increased height of the posterior wall relative to the height of the adjacent vertebra is a fundamental sign. This characteristic feature distinguishes this lesion from fractures due to compression mechanisms, in which the height of the posterior wall is diminished.

Conversely, the anterior wall can show a slight wedge compression secondary to a mechanism of intrinsic compression.

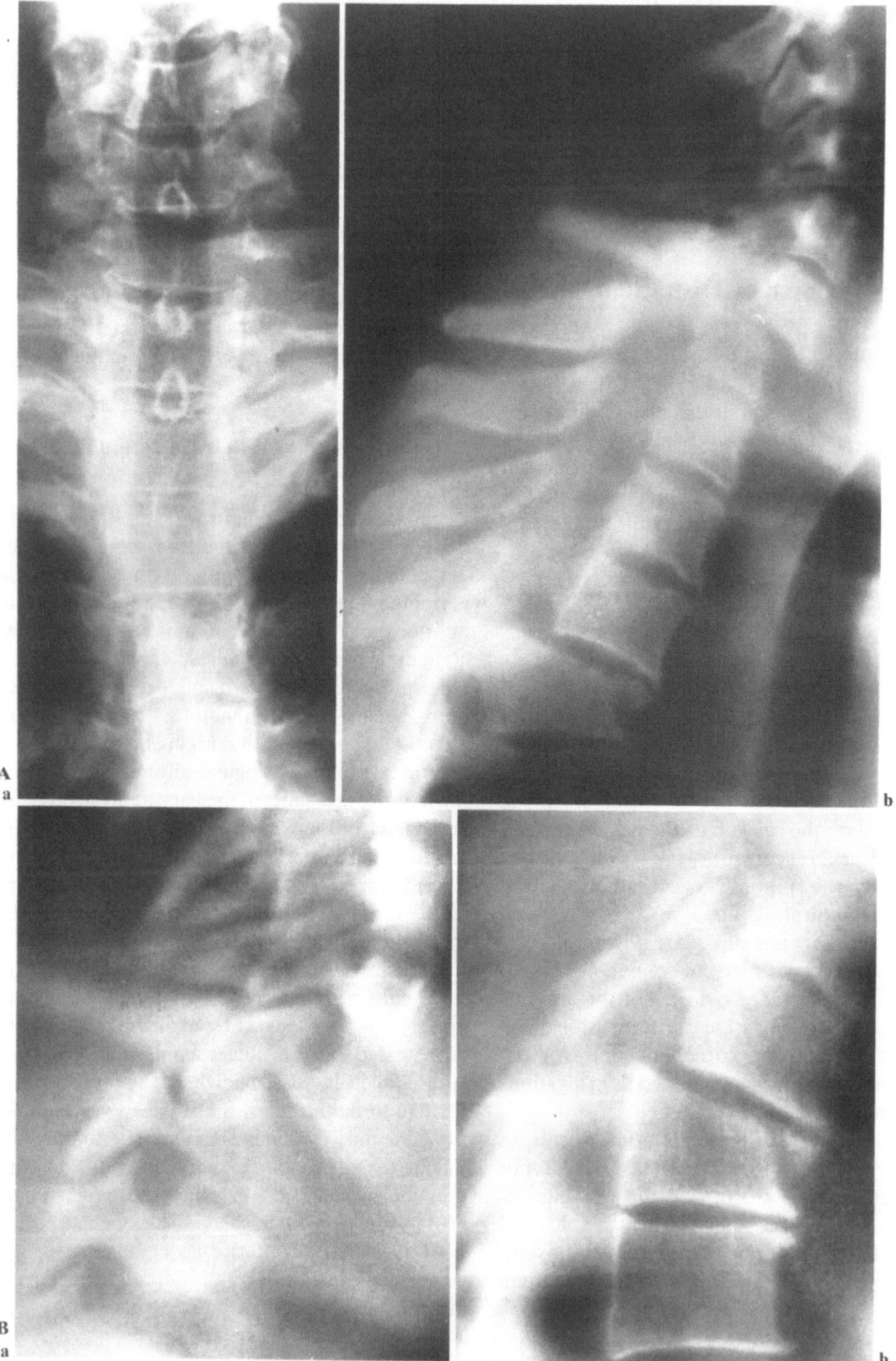

A
a
b
B
a
b Fig. 62 A, B

◁ **Fig. 62 A, B.** Luxations, C6–C7 and T3–T4, with paraplegia at level C7.
A Frontal and tomographic lateral views. The positioning for the lateral projection with shifted shoulders provides a more homogeneous contrast and thus allows a global view of the lower cervical and upper thoracic spine.
B Tomographic detail showing the over the top luxation of C6–C7 **(a)** and the T3–T4 **(b)** luxation

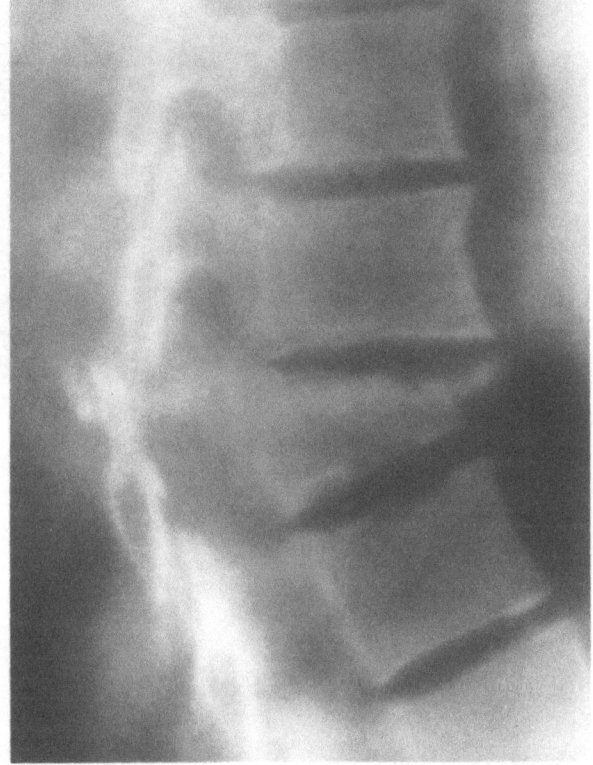

Fig. 63. Fracture-luxation of T8 caused by lesion sustained following compression in flexion. The patient was ejected from his car. There is complete paraplegia at the T8 level. The tomogram displays the luxation with fracture of the superior articular process and marked wedge compression of the T8 body

II. In Extension

1. Discoligamentous Lesions

The lesions are identical but there is no anterior marginal fracture. The diagnosis is made from the dynamic studies. The film taken during extension shows marked anterior gaping.

2. Bony Lesions

The radiologic sign of type II tear-drop fracture is the presence of an anterior corporeal fracture line, located on the lower end-plate and running obliquely down- and backward. The fracture line continues through the disk and disinserts the strong posterior longitudinal ligament. The injured vertebra undergoes retrolisthesis, which is seen as a backward shift of the posterior wall and posterior interarticular diastasis. In this case the lesion corresponds to an involvement of the anterior mobile spinal segment (Fig. 65).

Finally, the distraction lesions can be classified in the following way: they all belong to what we call group I, type A for the flexion mechanisms and to type B for the extension mechanisms.

B. Lesions Caused by Compression

The spine is continuously subjected to compression forces. Its equilibrium is assured by the state of preconstraint in the intervertebral disk and by the tension of the ligamentous and muscular structures.

There are, schematically, two types of compression forces. One of them is intrinsic and constituted by the weight of the body, which is distributed over all the vertebrae. In the upright position the constraints thus exerted increase from the axis to the 5th lumbar vertebra. The other type of force is of extrinsic origin, and appears as an exterior force that is applied in the axial direction. The direction of these forces is usually vertical due to the effect of the law of gravity, for example when something falls on the vertex or on the back.

In some circumstances, for example in road accidents, this force can have a horizontal direction. This is the case for a cyclist who runs into a tree with his head down. For classification purposes, axial compression forces are those that are

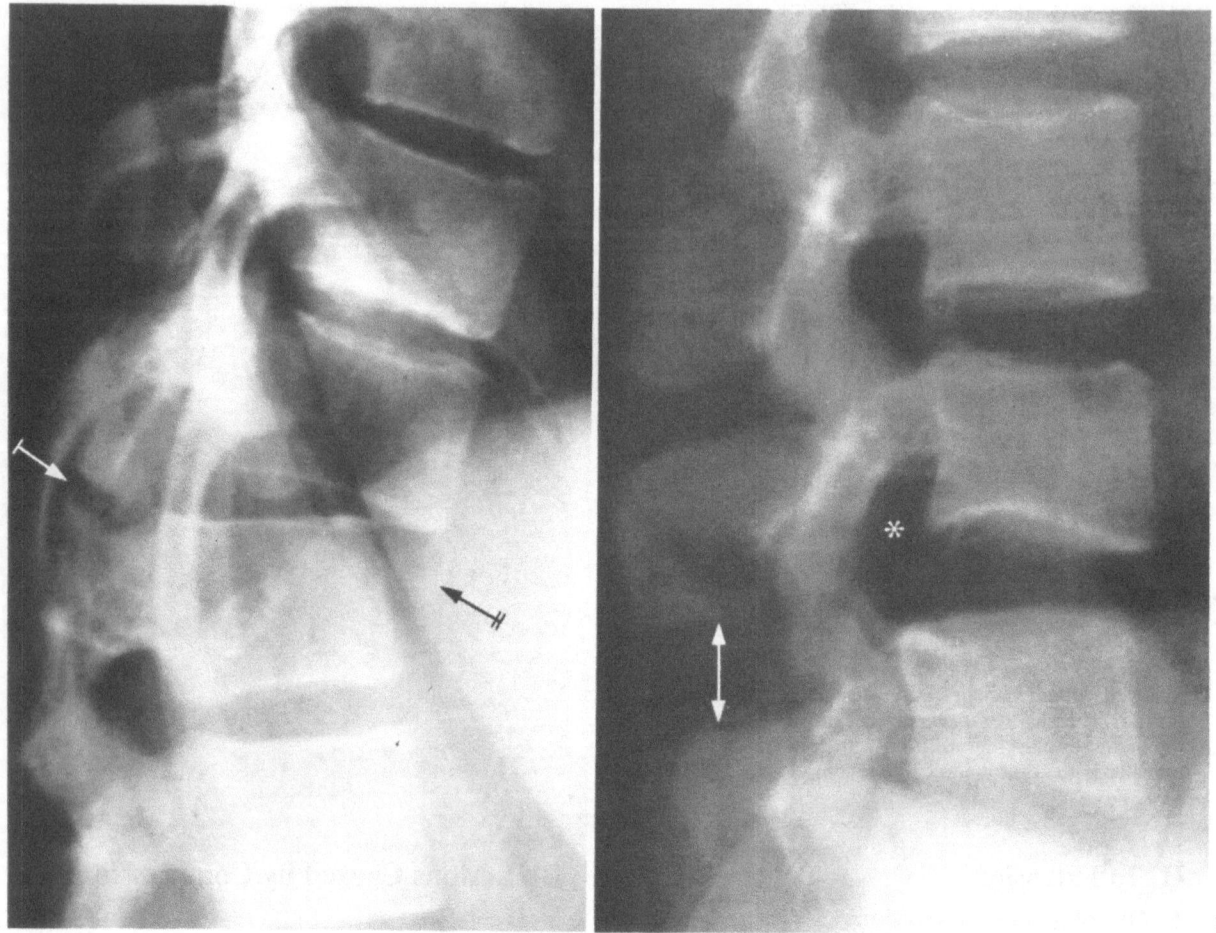

a   b

Fig. 64a, b. Distraction in flexion lesions. Multiple lesions following a traffic accident in a passenger who was ejected from the car although he had fastened his seat belt. Complete paraplegia at T12 level. **a** on the top luxation of T12–L1. The inferior articular process of T12 is aligned with the superior articular process of L1 (⊢→) and avulsion of an anterosuperior corner of L1 has occurred (⊬→). **b** L4–L5 subluxation or severe sprain, seen 10 days after the injury. The interspinous distance (↔) and the L4–L5 foramina (*) have become widened

applied more or less perpendicular to the direction of the vertebral plates, as opposed to shearing forces, which are transmitted parallel to these plates.

In normal functioning conditions of the vertebral spine the intrinsic compression forces resolve into three reaction forces, which ensure the equilibrium of the whole set: a first, axial force, acting perpendicular to the vertebral plate; a second, tangential force, acting in a direction parallel to the same plate; and a bending moment, the value of which is equivalent to that of the acting force multiplied by the distance separating the site of action from the site of application of the force.

The effect of extrinsic compression forces action depends on the position of the spine. During extension they act upon the posterior, vertebral arch. During flexion the repercussions are mainly on the vertebral body. The different vectorial components then act in the following ways. The axial force causes corporeal compressions and fractures: the tangential force makes antelisthesis likely; and the bending moment causes sprains or posterior interapophyseal luxations.

In the neutral position it can be expected that the forces will be distributed evenly over the three pillars, i.e., the anterior column and the two posterior articular columns.

I. In Flexion

The lesions always begin on the vertebral body. Sometimes they consist in partial or total compression, sometimes in a frontal or sagittal vertical fracture (Fig. 66).

Their site is usually the upper end-plate, except in the case of mechanisms with reverse compression such as occur in diving, in which case they involve the lower end-plate. Displacements always occur in the following way: the intact vertebral plate is displaced foward relative to the injured plate.

1. Partial or Anterior Wedge Compression

This lesion spares the posterior wall. Usually this mechanism is accompanied by hyperflexion, so that signs of benign or severe posterior sprain should be searched for, especially at the level of the cervical spine.

If not reduced this lesion causes kyphosis, which in association with disk degeneration produces posterior articular dysfunction; this in turn can lead to posterior arthrosis in the thoracolumbar segment and to subluxation or luxation in the cervical segment.

In this event there is also anterior displacement of the spinal segment above.

2. Global Compression

Total compression involves the posterior wall and can be symmetrical or asymmetrical. There is usually no posterior ligamentous instability, but there is a vertical rupture in the continuity, usually in the lamina, which explains the horizontal bursting of the vertebra.

In the light of these data it can be said that lesions of the posterior arch associated with vertebral compressions are divided into ligamentous lesions in partial wedge compression, which are the more likely when the compression is anterior, and fracture of the posterior arch in the case of global compression.

3. Body Fractures

Unlike the previous lesions, body fractures do not cause bone instability.

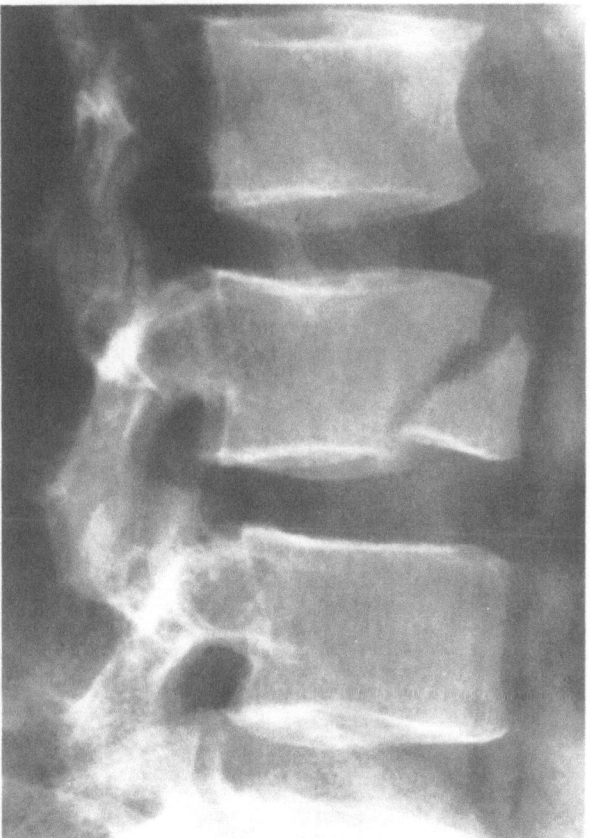

Fig. 65. Tear-drop fracture of L3 with disinsertion of the antero-inferior corner of L3 by an oblique downward and backward fracture line. The corner remains joined to the disk and the vertebra below. There is discrete retrolysthesis of L3 on L4. The lesion was caused by a backward fall with hyperextension.

4. Tear-Drop Fracture Type I

This type of tear-drop fracture is not caused by distraction, but by reversed compression. The mechanism corresponds to a force exerted from above downward, as in diving, or from below upward, as in the case of an automobile accident during which the driver hits roof of his car (Figs. 67 and 68).

In this event it is always the lower end-plate that is injured and the direction of the fracture line or of the wedge compression is reversed, i. e., no longer obliquely downward and forward, but obliquely downward and backward.

In the same way, the displacement relative to the intact segment is anterior.

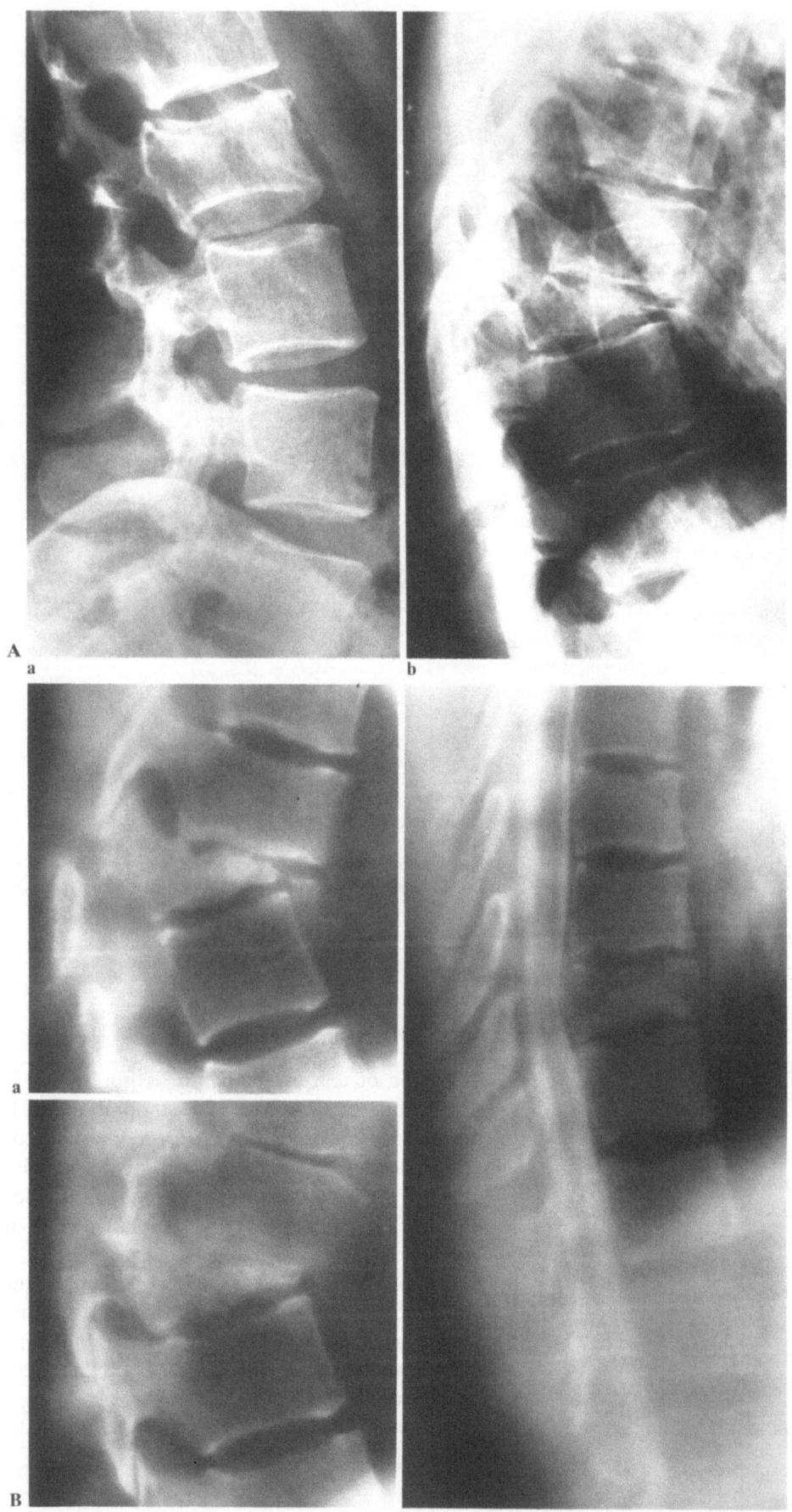

Fig. 66 A, B

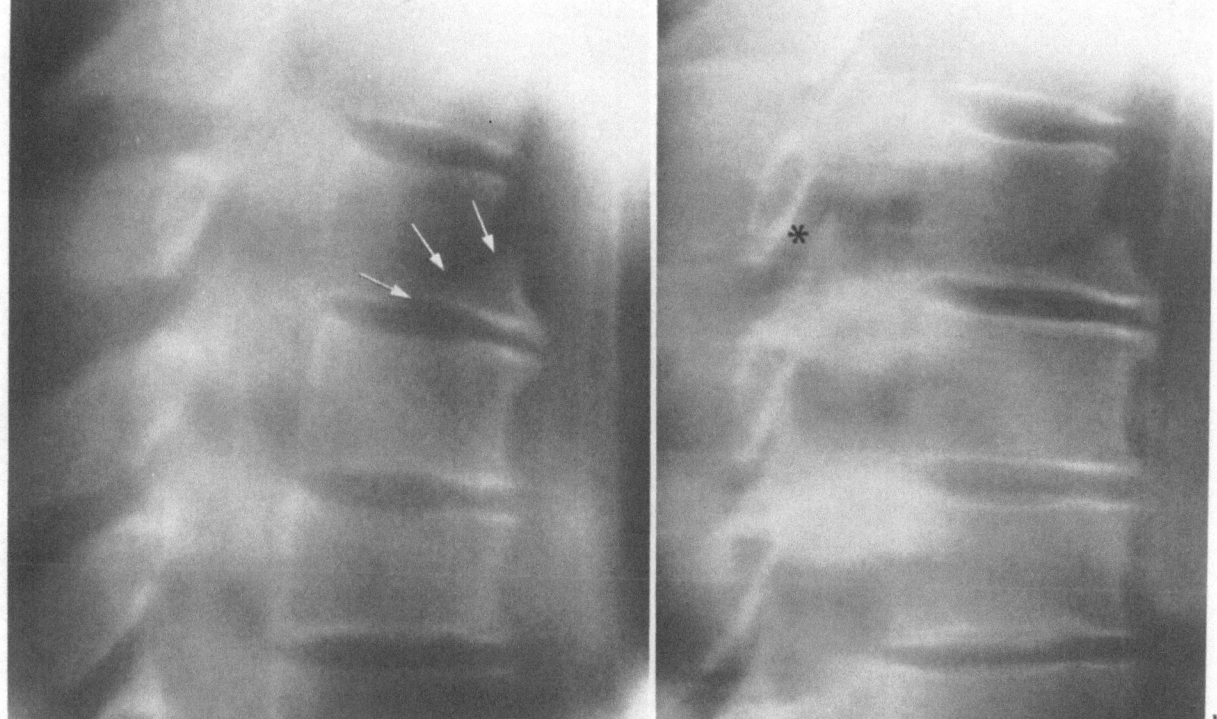

Fig. 67 a, b

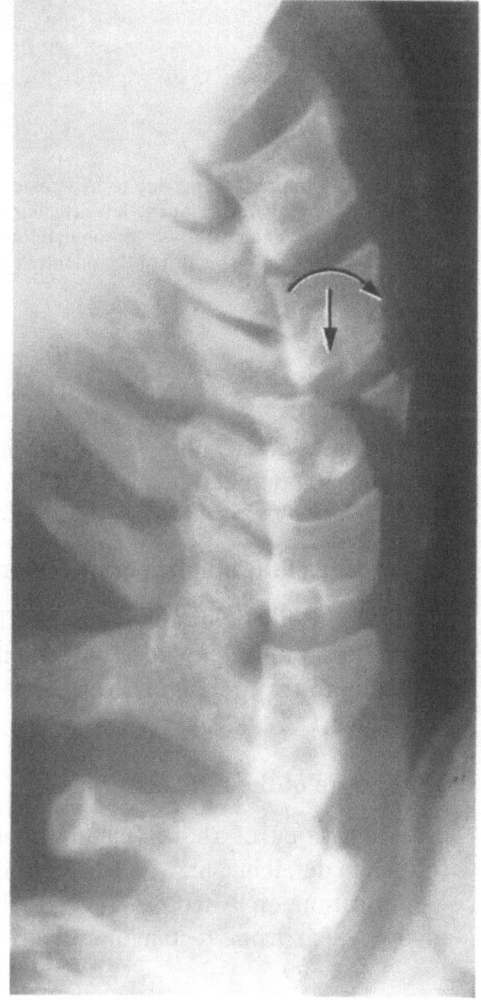

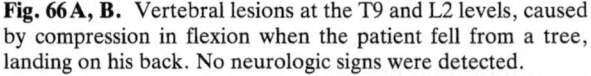

Fig. 66 A, B. Vertebral lesions at the T9 and L2 levels, caused by compression in flexion when the patient fell from a tree, landing on his back. No neurologic signs were detected.
A a Compression of the L2 body, with a slight backward displacement of the superior part of the posterior wall into the vertebral canal; **b** compression of T9 which is reduced to a corner with posterior base.
B The lamina of T9 is fractured, but the over- and underlying posterior interarticular connections are spared **(a, b)**. The myelography performed after reduction shows a moderate cord compression in T9 and a fracture of the spinous process of T9 **(c)**

Fig. 67 a, b. Tear-drop fracture of T4 caused by a road injury and followed by complete flaccid paraplegia at clinical level T4. Note avulsion of the anteroinferior corner of the vertebral plate of T4, which remains attached to the superior vertebral plate of the underlying vertebra (arrows) **(a)** and T4–T5 retrolisthesis, accompanied by posterior interarticular gaping (*) **(b)**

Fig. 68. Tear-drop fracture type I, caused by a reversed compression lesion. The figure is presented in the position of the injury

Fig. 68

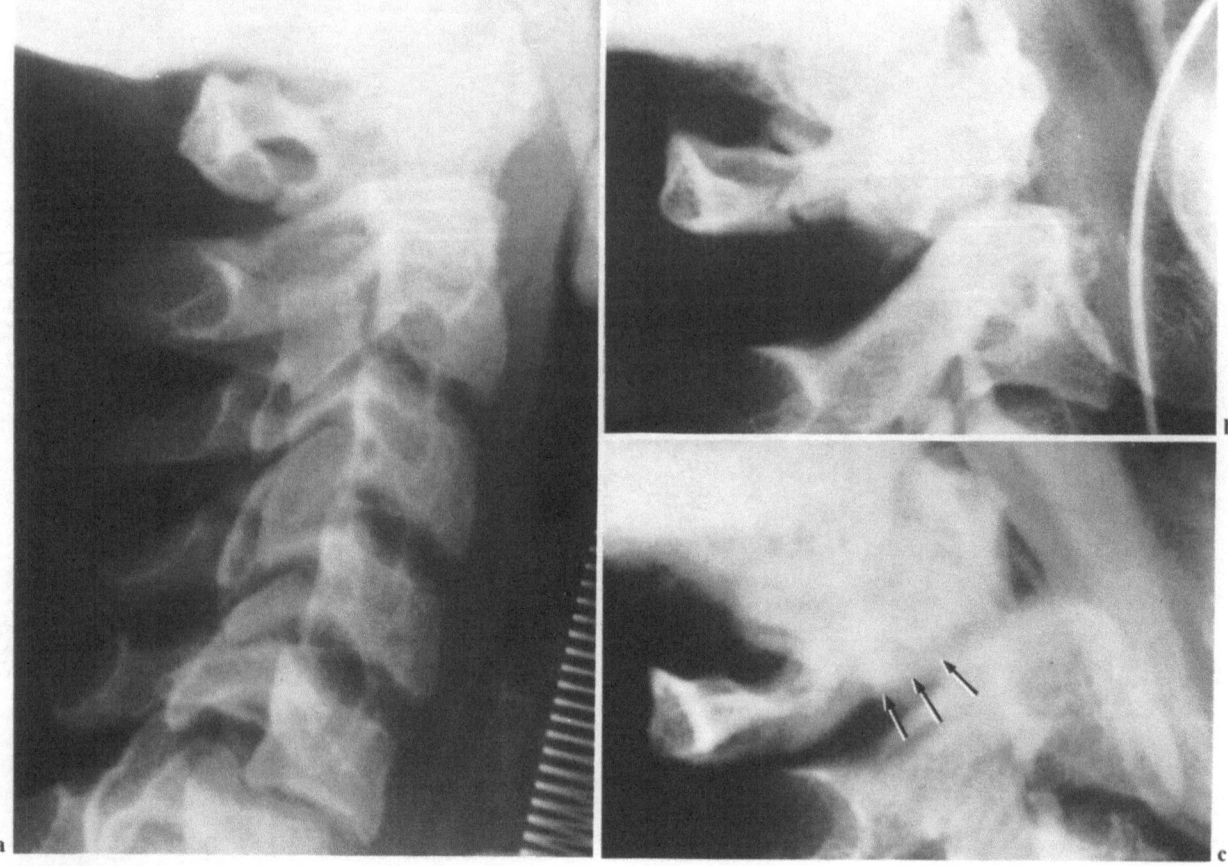

Fig. 69a–c. Multiple lesions due to hyperextension-compression: **a** fracture-separation of the left articular process of C5, causing lateralized antelisthesis syndrome; **b** fracture of the left posterior arch of C1; **c** fracture of the odontoid process leading to posterior displacement *(arrow)*. This case should be compared with the one illustrated in Fig. 28 (multiple lesions resulting from hyperextension-distraction)

II. In Extension

The main lesions resulting from compression during extension detailed below.

1. Fracture of the Spinous Processes and Laminae

The fracture line is usually vertical. The dynamic studies do not give evidence of instability; in particular there are no signs of severe posterior sprain.

2. Fracture of the Articular Pillars

The semiology of these fractures has been described in detail in Chap. 2. The main signs are the identification on a frontal view of the articular pillar, which from rectangular tends to become square with hypervisibility of the sub- and/or suprajacent articular interspaces. On the lateral view the posterior articular columns are seen to be misaligned, without antelisthesis of the corresponding vertebral body.

Disinsertion of the articular pillar occurs with a double fracture, one anterior and pedicular, usually visible on an oblique projection, and the other posterior and laminar; it can be overlooked on standard films but is shown on tomograms. The lesion is usually unilateral, since it occurs most often when the spine is in lateral flexion.

3. Fracture of the Pedicles

Fractures of the pedicles cause disinsertion of the posterior vertebral arch. This has a tendency to shift forward, producing a monocorporeal antelis-

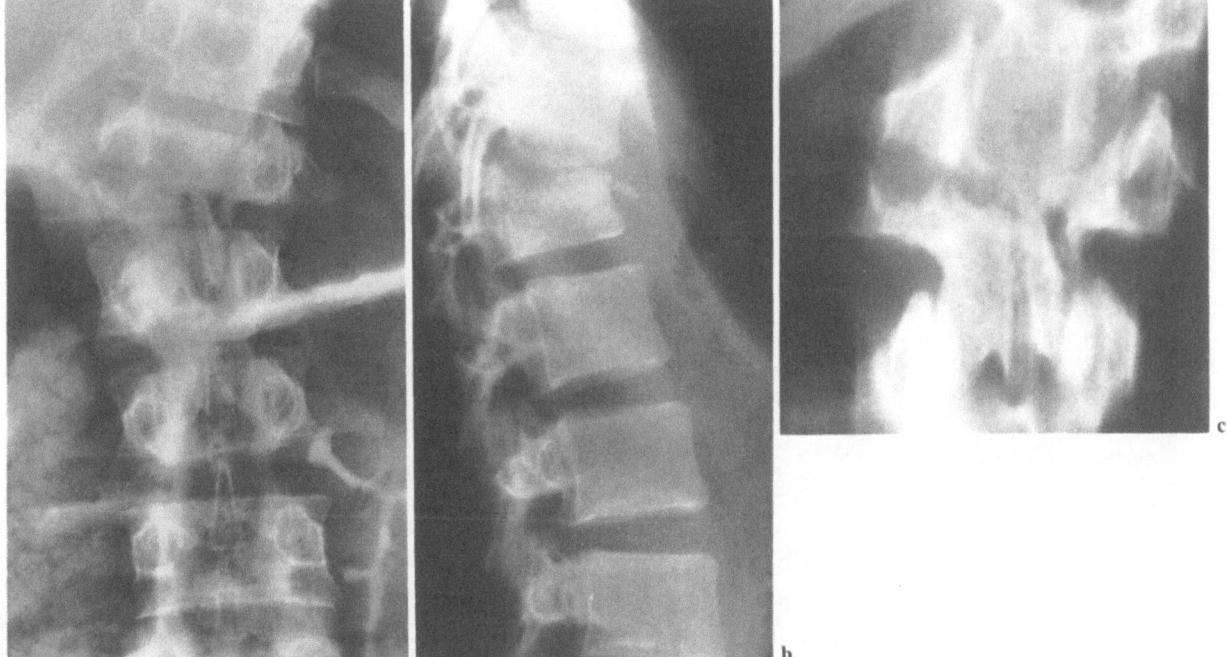

Fig. 70 a–c. Fracture of L1 caused by rotation mechanisms in a traffic accident during which the driver was ejected. No neurologic signs were detected: **a** frontal view, **b** lateral view, **c** tomogram of the posterior arch. The horizontal fracture line passes through the transverse process, the articular pillar and the pedicle on the right, and on the left vertical fracture line passes through the pars interarticularis. Compare this lesion with that shown in Fig. 57 (seat-belt fracture)

thesis, in contrast to the total antelisthesis caused by luxations and fractures of the articular processes.

C. Lesions Caused by Rotation

Lesions due to rotation occur almost only in the cervical and lumbar segments. Since it is protected by the rib cage the thoracic spine is only very exceptionally exposed to torsion.

The cervico-occipital joint is affected by two types of lesions, depending on the situation of the rotation axis. In the first case the pivot of rotation is situated to the front and passes through the vertebral body, or more generally through the intervertebral disk. In the second case the rotation pivot is situated at the back on a posterior interapophyseal column of the right or the left. Due to the difference in the orientation of the posterior articular facets of the cervical and lumbar vertebrae, the lesions are not the same. Taking into account this

anatomical peculiarity we can, however, affirm that the osteoligamentous changes involve predominantly the posterior vertebral arch.

I. Cervical Segment

The purest lesion is unilateral posterior interapophyseal luxation, which is due to the presence of a posterior rotation pivot centered on the contralateral articular pillar. Bone lesions, such as fracture of the superior and/or inferior articular process, are sometimes associated. Radiologically the lesion is evidenced by a lateralized antelisthesis, as described in Chap. 2. Anteriorly, on the vertebral body one should search for lesions of the antirotatory rails, i. e., the uncinate processes. The severity of the anterior discoligamentous changes determines the extent to which this type of lesion is stable.

Besides unilateral luxation with or without articular lesions, we recognize in this type of mechanism the fracture-separation of the articular pillar,

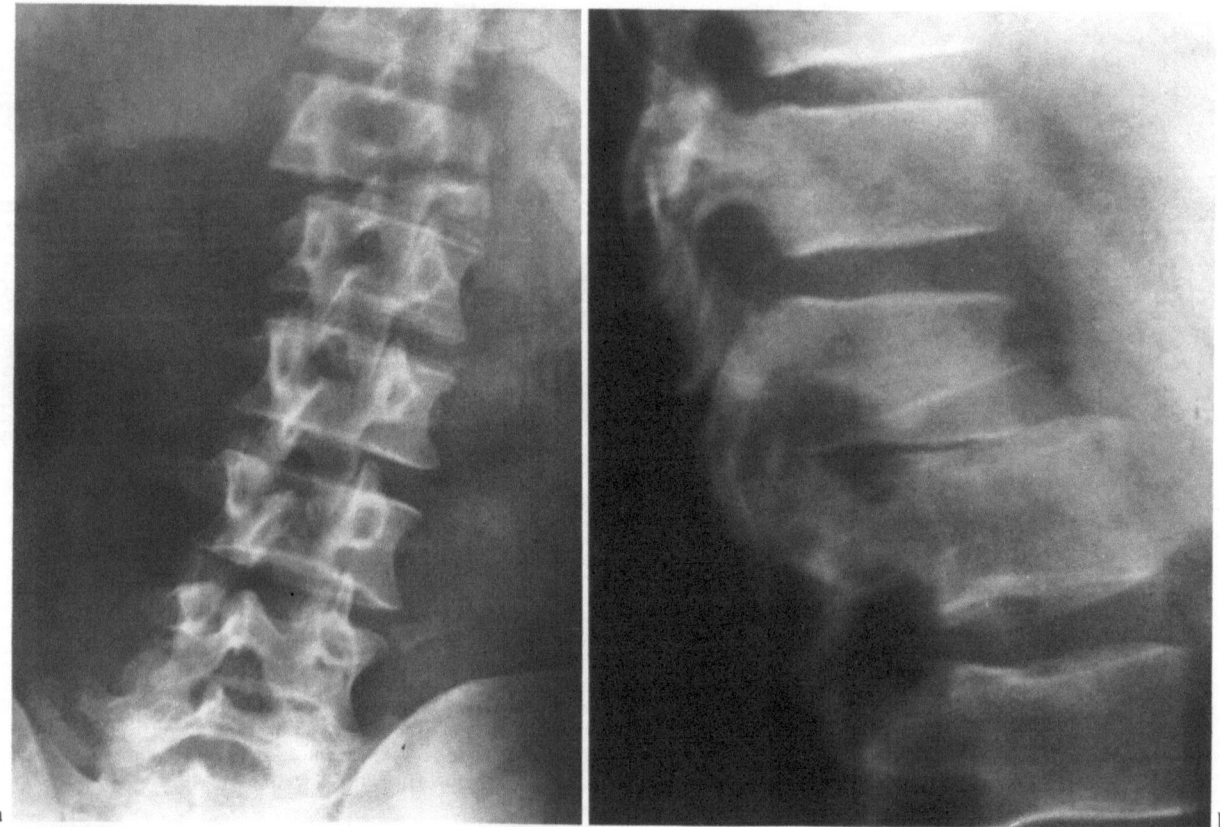

Fig. 71a, b

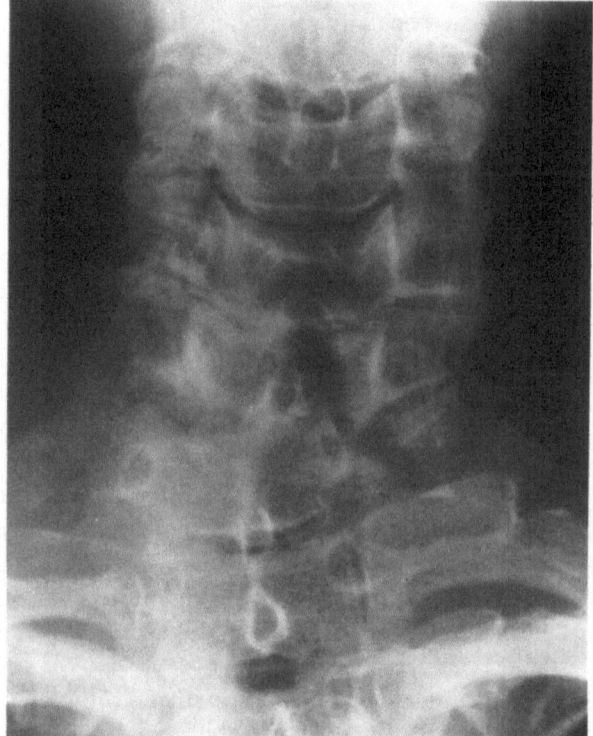

Fig. 71a, b. Fracture of T12 caused by transverse shearing in a bicycle rider run over by a car. No immediate neurologic signs were detected. A secondary occurrence was monoparesis of the left lower limb. Frontal (**a**) and lateral (**b**) views show the disalignment in T12–L1. Posterolateral displacement of the lumbar segment has resulted from the shearing mechanism

Fig. 72. C6–C7 fracture-luxation dislocation originally unnoticed in a patient with acute alcoholism, and discovered 24 h after occurrence

Fig. 72

which is also evidenced radiologically by lateralized antelisthesis. In this syndrome it is mainly unilateral uncovertebral gaping that gives evidence of a torsion-rotation movement.

II. Lumbar Segment

In Chap. 1 we saw that the natural center of the rotation movements is situated on the side of the spinous process and that it exerts constant constraint on the intervertebral disk. The disk is particularly susceptible to torsion movements, so that its involvement is almost constant. With reference to the posterior vertebral arch, the lesions consist of fractures of the isthmus on the same side as the rotation pivot, and of posterior interapophyseal gaping of the transverse type on the opposite side. Involvement of the transverse processes is almost constant, and predominates on the contralateral side to the rotation axis. In this case the fracture line is always horizontal, in contrast to what occurs with fractures of the transverse process due to hyperflexion or hyperextension, when the fracture line is more likely to be vertical, usually connected with excessive traction of the psoas muscle (Fig. 70).

D. Lesions Caused by Shearing Movements

Lesions caused by shearing are always related to direct traumas. This basic fact explains why in this type of trauma the musculovertebral lesions are always located opposite to the point of impact.

They usually result from very violent traumas, which dislocate the vertebral column into two distinct blocks. Because of the damage and the unavoidable fracture-displacements, the lesions caused by shearing movements are highly neurotoxic and particularly unstable. There are no specific lesions with this type of mechanism, but there are nevertheless some characteristic features, i.e., both the bony and the discoligamentous or even muscular lesions are all located in the same plane, which is the action line of the forces. This fracture plane is usually horizontal following posteroanterior impacts and oblique after transverse impacts. In this regard it can be compared to a CHANCE's fracture, although there is the following fundamental difference: a CHANCE's fracture affects the bone exclusively, while a fracture caused by shearing forces is mixed, so that the lesions look as though they result from a hatchet blow delivered without discrimination as to the different structures encountered (Figs. 71 and 72).

Fracture displacements are frequent and follow the rule of translation. But on account of the extreme instability of the lesions, the direction of the displacements has no informative value; any inopportune maneuver can change the orientation of the displacement.

The neurotoxicity of this type of lesions is so extreme that the neurologic damage caused is usually irreversible. In our opinion these lesions require internal fixation, i.e., surgery (screwed plaque, HARRINGTON's device, etc.) to permit nursing and to avoid the formation of scabs, an unavoidable complication of orthopedic treatment with plaster appliances due to sensory disturbances.

Conclusions

At the end of this work aimed at an analytic and comprehensive study of vertebral traumas we are aware that conventional radiographic investigation remains vastly inadequate. Provided that a rigorous analysis is made, however, the great majority of therapeutic problems can be solved. This is particularly true for the nonneurologic traumatic spine. CT investigations certainly provide additional data by displaying the bone lesions in more detail, thanks to the third dimension. To our knowledge, however, they do not seem to solve the problem of the diagnosis of discoligamentous lesions any differently than does conventional radiography, i.e., by studying the displacements. Therefore in our opinion scanography is still not sufficiently informative for examination of the neurologic traumatic spine.

How can we indeed consider the presence of an intracanalar bone fragment responsible for the neurologic signs presented by an injured patient when in similar conditions and with equivalent data another patient emerges unscathed from a vertebral trauma? Such findings have been commonly recorded in myelographies and are in fact only a factor of risk. For our part we believe that the differentiation power of CT is still insufficient insofar as the structures of the central nervous system are concerned. Perhaps RMN will solve the problem of the etiology of neurologic damage to the spine in the near future, by displaying edema, attrition, hematoma, medullary section, or just the genuine pathogenicity of medullary compression.

References

Anderson LD, D'Alonzo RT (1974) Fractures of the odontoid process of the axis. J Bone Joint Surg [Am] 56:1664–1674

Aufdermaur M (1974) Spinal injuries in juveniles necropsy; findings in 12 cases. J Bone Joint Surg [Br] 56:513–519

Babin E, Babin SR (1981) Lésions traumatiques du rachis cervical moyen et inférieur. Traumatic lesions of the middle and lower cervical spine. Radiologie J CEPUR 1:111–122

Baldini G, Guareschi B (1958) Observations sur l'examen radiologique fonctionnel du rachis cervical. Technique d'examen. Minerva Med 49:117–122

Balmary G, Gabet F, Philandrianos G (1981) Une lésion bipolaire du rachis cervical. J Traumatologie 2:83–86

Barcat E, Rigault P, Padovani JP, Martin P (1975) Fractures et luxations du rachis cervical chez l'enfant. Ann Chir Inf 17:197–212

Beatson TR (1963) Fractures and dislocations of the cervical spine. J Bone Joint Surg [Br] 45:21–34

Bensahel H (1968) Luxations et fractures du rachis cervical chez l'enfant. Rev Chir Orthop 54:765–780

Bisserie M (1978) Etude anatomique et physio-pathologique du grand ligament vertébral commun postérieur. Thesis, Paris, Université René Descartes (Cochin)

Blery M, Prebay TH (1978) Les fractures du rachis de l'adulte en traumatologie. Cours de Perfectionnement Post-Universitaire

Blery M, Chagnon S, Balmary G (1981) Les entorses graves du rachis cervical chez l'adulte. J Traumatologie 3:125–132

Bleynie JF (1977) Fractures des pédicules de l'axis (à propos de 44 cas). Thèse médecine, Paris

Boger D, Ralls PW (1981) New traction device for radiography of the lower cervical spine. AJR 137:1202–1204

Botton G (de) (1975) Fracture de l'apophyse odontoïde; essai d'analyse et de classification sur 34 cas. Déductions thérapeutiques. Medical thesis, Paris

Braakman R, Penning L (1968) The hyperflexion sprain of the cervical spine. Radiol Chir Biol 37:309–320

Braakman R, Penning L (1971) Injuries of the cervical spine. Excerpta Medica, Amsterdam

Caffiniere JY, Seringe R, Roy-Camille R, Saillant G (1972) Etude physio-pathologique des lésions ligamentaires graves dans les traumatismes de la charnière occipito-rachidienne. Rev Chir Orthop 58:11–19

Calenoll LC, Chessare JW, Rogers LF, Toerge J, Rosen JS (1978) Multiple level spinal injuries: importance of early recognition. AJR 130:665–669

Carlioz H, Dubousset J (1973) Les instabilités entre atlas et axis chez l'enfant. Rev Chir Orthop 59:291–301

Cattel JS, Filtzer PL (1965) Pseudoluxation and other normal variation in the cervical spine in children. J Bone Joint Surg [Am] 47:1295–1309

Chance GO (1948) Note on a type of flexion fracture of the spine. Br J Radiol 21:452–453

Clark WM, Gehweiler JA, Laib R (1979) Twelve significant signs of cervical spine trauma. Skeletal Radiol 3:201–205

Daffner RH (1967) Pseudofracture of the dens: Mach bands. AJR 128:607

Dany A, Tasson P, Treves R, Ravon R, Bokor J (1977) Complete bilateral post-traumatic-dislocation L4–L5 without fracture. Sem Hop Paris 53:437–439

De Botton G (1975) Les fractures de l'apophyse odontoïde. Essai de classification et d'analyse sur 34 cas. Déduction thérapeutique. Medical thesis, Paris

Decoulx P (1973) Mobilités du rachis cervical. Nouv Presse Med 2:657–659

Delahaye RP, Metges PJ (1976) Aspects radiologiques des fractures du rachis. In: Radiodiagnostic II/3, Paris (Encycl Med Chir, P31040, B-10 and B-20)

Dewey P, Browne PS (1968) Fracture-dislocation of the lumbosacral spine with cauda equina lesion. Report of two cases. J Bone Joint Surg [Br] 50:635–638

Dorland P, Fremont-Parker J, Perez J (1958) Techniques d'examen radiologique de l'arc postérieur des vertèbres cervico-dorsales. J Radiol 39:509–519

Effendi B, Roy D, Cornish B, Dussault RG, Laurin CA (1981) Fractures of the ring of the axis. J Bone Joint Surg [Br] 63:319–327

Elliot JM Jr, Rogers LF, Wissinger JP, Lee JF (1972) The hangman's fracture. Radiology 104:303–307

Epstein BS (1976) The spine. A radiological text and atlas. Lea & Febiger, Philadelphia

Fielding JW (1964) Mobilité normale et anormale de la colonne cervicale depuis la deuxième vertèbre cervicale jusqu'à la septième étudiée en radio-cinéma. J Bone Joint Surg [Am] 46:1779–1781

Filipe G, Berges O, Lebard JP, Carlioz H (1982) Intabilités post traumatiques entre l'atlas et l'axis chez l'enfant. A propos de 5 observations. Rev Chir Orthop 68:461–469

Fischer L, Neidhardt JH, Dechaume M, Bochu M (1969a) Intérêt radiologique du disque inter-axo-odontoïdien. Rev Radiol 50:847–849

Fischer L, Neidhardt JH, Gerentes R, Spay G (1969b) Structure macroscopique de l'apophyse odontoïde d'après l'étude anatomo-radiologique. Lyon Med 222:433–440

Fischer L, Texier D'Arnoult A (1970) Fractures de l'apophyse odontoïde de l'axis chez l'adulte. Cah Med Lyonnais 46:1283–1308

Francis WR, Fielding JW, Hawkins RJ, Pepin J, Hensinger R (1981) Traumatic spondylolisthésis of the axis. J Bone Joint Surg [Br] 63:313–318

Gehweiler JA, Clark WM, Schaaf RE, Powers B, Miller MD (1979) Cervical spine trauma: the common combined conditions. Radiology 130:77–86

Gehweiler JA, Osborne RL, Becker RF (1980) The radiology of vertebral trauma. Saunders, Philadelphia

Gerlock AJ, Kirchner SG, Heller RM, Kaye JJ (1978) The cervical spine in trauma. Saunders, Philadelphia

Gouraud D (1981) Etude radiologique de la stabilité du rachis cerical de l'enfant. Thesis, Paris

Grogono BJS (1954) Injuries of the atlas and the axis. J Bone Joint Surg [Am] 36:397–410

Harris JH Jr (1978) The radiology of acute cervical spine trauma. Williams & Wilkins, Baltimore

Haughton S (1866) On hanging, considered from a mechanical and physiological point of view. London, Edinburgh and Dublin Philosophical Magazine and Journal of Science 4th Series 32:23–34

Hohl M, Baker HR (1964) L'articulation atloïdo-axoïdienne. Etude anatomique et radiologique des mouvements normaux et anormaux. J Bone Joint Surg [Am] 46:1739–1752

Holdsworth FW (1963) Fractures, dislocations and fracture-dislocations of the spine. J Bone Joint Surg [Br] 45:6–20

Holdsworth F (1970) Fractures, dislocation, and fracture-dislocations of the spine. J Bone Joint Surg [Am] 52:1534–1551

Husby J, Sorensen KH (1974) Fracture of the odontoïd process of the axis. Acta Orthop Scand 45:182–192

Judet R, Judet J, Roy-Camille R, Zerah JC, Saillant G (1970) Fracture du rachis cervical: fracture-séparation du massif articulaire. Rev Chir Orthop 56:155–164

Juhl JH, Miller SM, Roberts GW (1962) Roentgenographic variations in the normal cervical spine. Radiology 78:591–597

Jung A, Kehr P (1970) Les traumatismes du rachis cervical avec lésions vasculaires. J Chir 99:127–144

Kauffer H, Hayes J (1966) Lumbar fracture-dislocation: A study of twenty one cases. J Bone Joint Surg [Am] 48:712–730

Lee C, Kim KS, Rogers LF (1982) Triangular cervical vertebral body fractures: Diagnostic significance. AJR 138:1123–1132

Locke GR, Gardner JI, van Epps EF (1966) Intervalle atlas-odontoïde chez l'enfant. Une étude basée sur 200 colonnes cervicales normales. AJR 97:135–140

Louis R (1977) Les théories de l'instabilité. Symposium SO.F.C.O.T. Rev Chir Orthop 63:423–425

Louis R (1979a) Traumatismes du rachis cervical. Entorses et hernies discale. Nouv Presse Med 8:1843–1849

Louis R (1979b) Traumatismes du rachis cervical. Fractures et luxations. Nouv Presse Med 8:1931–1937

Louis R, Goutallier D (1977) Fractures instables du rachis. Rev Chir Orthop 63:417–475

McCoy SH, Johnson KA (1976) Sagittal fracture of the cervical spine. J Trauma 16:310–312

Merle P, Geroget MM, Viallet JF (1970) Etude radiologique dynamique des rapports de l'atlas et de l'axis chez l'enfant. J Radiol 51:6–7, 373–377

Michel G (1977) Les fractures de l'apophyse odontoïde, étude clinique de 63 cas, étude expérimentale, déduction thérapeutique. Medical thesis, Paris-Ouest

Mourgues (de) G, Fischer L, Jarsaillon B, Machenaud A (1973) Fractures de l'arc postérieur de l'axis. Rev Chir Orthop 59:549–564

Mourgues (de) G, Fischer LP, Bejui J, Carret JP, Gonon GP (1981) Fractures de l'apophyse odontoïde (Dens) de l'axis. 102 cas sont 73 fractures récentes. Rev Chir Orthop 67/8:783–790

Naidich JB, Naidich TP, Garfein C, Liebeskind AL, Hyman RA (1977) The widened interspinous distance: a useful sign of anterior cervical dislocation in the supine frontal projection. Radiology 123:113–116

Newell RL (1977) Lumbosacral fracture-dislocation: a case managed conservatively, with return to heavy work. Injury 9:131–134

Norton WL (1962) Fractures and dislocations of the cervical spine. J Bone Joint Surg [Am] 44:115–132

Pennecot GF, Chadoutaud JC, Pouliquen F (1981) Traumatismes graves du rachis de l'enfant. Ann Chir 35/7:506–512

Penning L (1978) Normal movements of the cervical spine. AJR 130:317–326

Penning L (1980) Prevertebral hematoma in cervical spine injury: incidence and etiologie significance. Am J Neuroradiol 1:557–565

Pouliquen JC, Beneux J, Pennecot GF (1978) Le risque de déviation rachidienne évolutive dans les fractures et luxations du rachis chez l'enfant. Rev Chir Orthop 64:487–498

Ramadier JO, Aleon J-F, Servant S (1976) Les fractures de l'apophyse odontoïde, 94 cas dont 61 traités par àrthrodèse. Rev Chir Orthop 62:171–189

Raymond RD, Wheeler PS, Perovic M (1972) The lucent cleft, a new radiographic sign of cervical disc injury or disease. Clin Radiol 23:188–192

Richmann S, Friedmann RL (1954) Vertical fractures of cervical vertebral bodies. Radiology 62:536–542

Roaf R (1960) A study of the mechanics of spinal injuries. J Bone Joint Surg [Br] 42:810–823

Roberts A, Wickstrom J (1972) Pronostics of odontoid fractures. J Bone Joint Surg [Am] 54:1353

Roy-Camille R (1979) Rachis cervical traumatique non neurologique. Premières Journées d'Orthopédie de la Pitié. Masson, Paris, pp 1–154

Roy-Camille R (1980) Rachis dorso-lombaire traumatique non neurologique. Deuxièmes Journées d'Orthopédie de la Pitié. Masson, Paris, pp 3–152

Roy-Camille R (1982) Rachis traumatique neurologique. Troisièmes Journées d'Orthopédie de la Pitié. Masson, Paris, pp 151–205

Roy-Camille R, Caffiniere JY, Saillant G (1972) L'entorse grave de la charnière occipito-rachidienne existe-t-elle? Rev Chir Orthop 58:4–10

Roy-Camille R, de la Caffiniere JY, Saillant G (1973) Traumatismes du rachis cervical supérieur C1–C2. Masson, Paris

Roy-Camille R, Bertaux D, Saillant G (1977) Analyse anatomo-radiologique. Symposium SO.F.C.O.T. Rev Chir Orthop 63:419–422

Roy-Camille R, Bleynie JF, Saillant G, Judet TH (1979) Fracture de l'otontoïde associée à une fracture des pédicules de l'axis. A propos de 11 cas. Rev Chir Orthop 65:387–391

Roy-Camille R, Gagnon P, Catonne Y, Benazet JP (1980a) La luxation antéro-latérale du rachis lombo-sacré: une lésion rare. Rev Chir Orthop 66:105–109

Roy-Camille R, Saillant G, Judet TH, Botton G, Michel G (1980b) Eléments de pronostic des fractures de l'odontoïde. Rev Chir Orthop 66:183–186

Samberg LC (1975) Fracture-dislocation of the lumbosacral spine. A case report. J Bone Joint Surg [Am] 57:1007–1008

Schatzker J, Rorabeck CH, Waddell JP (1971) Fractures de l'apophyse odontoïde, Analyse de 37 cas. J Bone Joint Surg [Br] 53:392–405

Scher AT (1977) Unilateral locked facet in cervical spine injuries. AJR 129:45–48

Scher AT (1979) Anterior cervical subluxation: a instable position. AJR 133:275–280

Schneider RC, Kahn EA (1956) Chronic neurological sequelae of acute trauma to the spine and spinal cord. The significance of the acute flexion or "tear drop" fracture dislocation of the cervical spine. J Bone Joint Surg [Am] 38:985–997

Sherk HH (1975) Lesions of the atlas and axis. Clin Orthop 109:33–41

Swischuk LE (1977) Anterior displacement of C2 in children. Radiology 122:759–763

Taylor TKF, Nade S, Bannister JH (1976) Seat belt fractures of the cervical spine. J Bone Joint Surg [Br] 58:328–331

Thiebaut F, Wackenheim A, Vrousos C (1960) Etudes de la charnière cervico-occipitale. J Radiol 41:302–308

Vlahovitch B, Fuentes JM, Linonm DE (1974) Les fractures bipédiculaires de l'axis. Montpellier Chir 20:211–220

Wackenheim A (1968) Traumatismes indirects du rachis cervical (coup de fouet, coup du lapin, cisaillement). Whip lash injury ou syndrome cervical posttraumatique. Feuillets électro-radiol 45:1–12

Wackenheim A (1966) La ligne médiane de la charnière cervico-occipitale. Etude d'une ligne inter-vestibulaire. Sem Hop Paris 42:1448–1451

Wackenheim A, Lopez F (1969) Etude radiographique des mouvements de C1 et C2 lors de la flexion et de l'extension de la tête. J Belge Radiol 52:117–120

Wackenheim A, Dupuis M, Dosch JCl (1980) Un signe indirect de hernie discale cervicale. J Radiol 61:11, 683–687

Wackenheim A, Wiest-Million S (1981) L'image radiologique de l'espace rétro-pharyngien. Compression et déplacement de l'espace rétro-pharyngien par l'hématome des entorses graves et fractures du rachis cervical. J Radiol CEPUR 1:123–131

Webb JK, Broughton RBK, McSweeney T, Park WM (1976) Hidden flexion injury of the cervical spine. J Bone Joint Surg [Br] 58:322–327

Weir Don C (1975) Radiological signs of cervical injury. Clin Orthop 109:9–17

Whalen JP, Woodruff CL (1970) The cervical prevertebral fat stripe. A new aid in evaluating the cervical prevertebral soft tissue space. AJR 109:445–451

White AA, Panjabi M (1978) Clinical biomechanics of the spine. Lippincott, Philadelphia

White AA, Johnson RM, Panjabi MM, Southwick WO (1975) Biomechanical analysis of clinical stability in the cervical spine. Clin Orthop 109:85–96

Whitley JE, Forsyth HF (1960) The classification of cervical spine injuries. Radiology 83:633–644

Wood-Jones F (1913) The ideal lesion produced by judicial hanging. Lancet I:53

Zanca P, Lodmell EA (1951) Fracture of spinous processes: new sign for recognition of fractures of cervical and upper dorsal spinous processes. Radiology 56:427–429

Subject Index

Page references referring to figures are given in *italics*

Atlas of Pathological Computer Tomography

In 3 volumes

Volume 1: **A. Wackenheim, L. Jeanmart, A. L. Baert**
Craniocerebral Computer Tomography
Confrontations with Neuropathology

With collaboration of D. Baleriaux, D. Crolla, J. Dietemann, R. Dom,
J. Flament, N. Heldt, Y. Palmers, J. Termote
1980. 112 figures in 498 separate illustrations. X, 130 pages.
ISBN 3-540-09879-8

Volume 2: **A. L. Baert, A. Wackenheim, L. Jeanmart**
Abdominal Computer Tomography

With collaboration of G. Marchal, G. Wilms
1980. 315 figures in 585 separate illustrations. XI, 185 pages.
ISBN 3-540-10093-8

Volume 3: **L. Jeanmart, A. L. Baert, A. Wackenheim**
Computer Tomography of Neck, Chest, Spine, and Limbs
With the collaboration of M. Osteaux
With contributions by numerous experts
1983. 545 figures. XI, 194 pages. ISBN 3-540-11439-4

J. F. Bonneville, J. L. Dietemann

Radiology of the Sella Turcica

With the collaboration of J. C. Demandre, G. Didierlaurent, C. Edus,
P. Gresyk, M. Pion, N. Quantin, T. Taillard
Illustrations by M. Gaudron
Translation Reviewed by I. Moseley
With a Foreword by J. L. Vezina, a Preface by A. Wackenheim and a
Historical Review by J. Metzger
1981. 370 figures in 693 separate illustrations. XXII, 262 pages.
ISBN 3-540-10319-8

J. A. L. Bulcke, A. L. Baert

Clinical and Radiological Aspects of Myopathies

CT Scanning – EMG – Radioisotopes
1982. 151 figures, 30 tables. XI, 187 pages. ISBN 3-540-11443-2

J. Chermet, J. M. Bigot

Venography of the Inferior Vena Cava and Its Branches

Translated from the French by M.-T. Wackenheim
1980. 243 figures, in 323 separate illustrations, 5 tables. XI, 232 pages
ISBN 3-540-09905-0

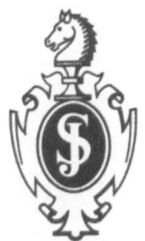

Springer-Verlag
Berlin
Heidelberg
New York
Tokyo

Contrast Media in Radiology

Appraisal and Prospects

First European Workshop - Proceedings -
Lyon 1981
Editor: **M. Amiel**
With the collaboration of J. F. Moreau
1982. 141 figures. XXI, 353 pages
ISBN 3-540-11534-X

P. Doury, Y. Dirheimer, S. Pattin

Algodystrophy

**Diagnosis and Therapy of a Frequent Disease of
the Locomotor Apparatus**

With a Foreword by J. Villiaumey
Translated from the French by
M.-T. Wackenheim
1981. 46 figures. XVI, 165 pages
ISBN 3-540-10624-3

A. Wackenheim

Radiodiagnosis of the
Vertebrae in Adults

125 Exercises for Students and Practitioners

1983. 250 figures. VI, 176 pages
(Exercises in Radiological Diagnosis)
ISBN 3-540-11681-8

Also available in German and French

A. Wackenheim

Cheirolumbar Dysostosis

**Developmental Brachycheiry and Stenosis of the
Bony Vertebral Lumbar Canal**

With collaboration of E. Babin, P. Bourjat,
E. Bromhorst, R. M. Kipper, R. Ludwiczak,
G. Vetter
Translated from the French by
M.-T. Wackenheim
1980. 39 figures, 85 tables. VII, 102 pages
ISBN 3-540-10371-6

A. Wackenheim, E. Babin

The Narrow Lumbar Canal

Radiologic Signs and Surgery

With a Foreword by L. Jeanmart
1980. 139 figures in 292 separate illustrations,
7 tables. XIII, 170 pages. ISBN 3-540-09443-1

Séries de diapositives

Anatomie normale du
médiastin en tomographie
computée

L. De Divano, M. Osteaux, T. Darras, L. Jeanmart

1983. 61 diapositives. Légendes en francais.
II, 9 pages. Livraison en classeur.
ISBN 3-540-92116-8

P. Peetrons, L. Jeanmart

Anatomie echographique de
l'abdomen supérieur: approche
de la pathologie par la
connaissance du normal

1983. 85 diapositives. Légendes en francais.
II, 10 pages. Livraison en classeur.
ISBN 3-540-92117-6

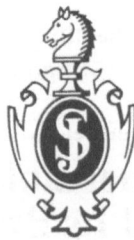

Springer-Verlag
Berlin Heidelberg New York Tokyo